Health of Nations

*An International Perspective on
U.S. Health Care Reform*

Health of Nations

*An International Perspective on
U.S. Health Care Reform*

THIRD EDITION

Laurene A. Graig

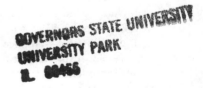

Congressional Quarterly, Inc.
Washington, D.C.

CQ Press
1414 22nd Street, N.W.
Washington, D.C. 20037
(202) 822-1475; (800) 638-1710

http://books.cq.com

Library of Congress Cataloging-in-Publication Data

Graig, Laurene A.
    Health of nations / Laurene A. Graig. — 3rd ed.
        p. cm.
    Includes bibliographical references and index.
    ISBN 1-56802-361-8 (hbk.). — ISBN 1-56802-360-X (pbk.)
    1. Medical care—Finance Case studies.   2. Medical care—United States—
Finance.   3. Insurance, Health—Government policy Case studies.
4. Insurance, Health—Government policy—United States.   5. Health care
reform—United States.   I. Title.
RA411.G68   1999
338.4′33621—DC21   99-23731
                                                             CIP

Contents

Tables and Figures

TABLES

FIGURES

Foreword

Health care is always among the top concerns of most Americans, and periodically the nation takes a long look at our health care system and asks how we might make it better. The reasons for this are simple, even if the solutions are not: the ranks of those without health insurance grow by a million per year. The percentage of Americans getting health insurance through an employer is steadily shrinking. The cost of individual health insurance is beyond the means of too many people. And more recently, people are chafing at the restrictions of managed care and are asking government to help protect their rights. There is little debate over whether we have the highest quality health care system in the world—the pervasive question is how to extend its benefits to more of our people.

In the third edition of *Health of Nations,* Laurene Graig has shown us how six nations—very different in their philosophies and cultures—are tackling similar nationwide health care dilemmas of balancing costs, quality, and access to care. She points out that all the countries she has studied have moved toward a more cost-conscious model of care. But, it is important to note, she demonstrates how nations with a history of providing health care to all of their citizens have retained universal access even as they institute American-inspired measures to control costs. These two goals—access for all and affordable care—clearly are not at odds and both can effectively be achieved.

It is clear that new opportunities for meaningful change of our health care system will arise again soon, making this insight especially timely. In considering health care reform, many Americans say that our country is unique, our health care needs are different from those of other countries, and for these reasons we need distinctly American solutions. Although there is certainly some truth to these sentiments, it is clear that the United States can learn a great deal from other nations. We must remember that America is a nation of immigrants who have brought the wisdom of experience from their lands of origin and, in the process, strengthened our country. Considering how insignificant international borders are becoming in so many aspects of our society, it would be shortsighted to reject health care lessons and solutions simply because they come from outside our boundaries.

Americans are also clear that they want to be able to retain those features they hold most dear, whether it is autonomy for physicians, choice of provider for patients, or the opportunity for health care providers to make a profit. Our solutions will, in the end, be uniquely American. But let us hope that, in devising our solutions, we take full advantage of the experience of other nations who have been down the same road.

I commend Laurene Graig for this helpful and hopeful work—and Watson Wyatt for sponsoring it. All of us involved in creating an improved health care system will learn from this detailed analysis. We need to understand the fundamental societal issues that have influenced the development of health care solutions in our country and in other nations. And we need to understand the experiences of other health care systems as we work to craft a health care system that will serve all Americans for years to come.

—Sen. John D. Rockefeller IV

Preface

In contrast to some public policy issues, health care is not an abstract concept. It is rather an issue that has direct impact on each and every American. In the early 1990s, a consensus emerged that America's costly and fragmented health care system fell short of the mark.

The 1992 presidential election was the first in almost three decades in which health care was a prominent issue. The debate focused not on whether change was needed in the health care system but instead on what the scope of that change should be. President George Bush advocated incremental change and tinkering around the edges. His challenger, Bill Clinton, called for universal coverage through a complete overhaul of the U.S. health care system—which amounted to one-seventh of the nation's economy. That was the situation when the second edition of *Health of Nations* was published.

What a difference six years makes. The Clinton administration's health reform proposal never saw the legislative light of day, and incremental measures have filled the policy void created by the failed attempt at major health care reform. At the same time, the health care market in the United States has been transformed by the widespread adoption of managed care arrangements. Health care did not even make it into the top tier of issues of concern to voters during the 1998 congressional elections, despite the fact that the number of uninsured Americans has increased at the rate of nearly one million a year since the Clinton proposal was crafted. The steady growth in the ranks of the uninsured has occurred despite a thriving economy and historically low rates of unemployment. Even in this positive economic environment, there has been a near deafening silence on the issue of devising ways to cover the uninsured. The focus of legislative efforts has shifted; Clinton's mantra of "health security for all" has been replaced by a widespread demand for higher quality and improved access to services—falling under the broad rubric of patients' rights—for those who already have insurance coverage.

As the analysis in this book makes clear, every health care system has shortcomings and no ideal system exists. The U.S. health care system is one of the most technically advanced in the world, but as a system of voluntary insurance coverage it leaves a larger share of its population without coverage while spending far more on health care than any other industrialized nation.

Whether the United States should try to address these problems by adopting some form of national health insurance has resurfaced sporadically as a public policy issue for more than forty years. The endurance of national health insurance as an issue is evidence of significant interest in the concept if not strong support for it. If support does reach critical mass, and if a system of national health insurance is considered as a serious option for reform, other industrialized nations' systems can serve as guides for the development of an American national health insurance system. As this book reveals, different models have operated around the world for many years and provide a wealth of experience from which the United States can draw. Compelling evidence from Europe, Japan, and Canada indicates that it is possible to maintain a system of universal health insurance in which premiums are related to individuals' incomes and not to their risk status, and that costs can be controlled by one or several powerful health care purchasers—whether governmental, such as provincial governments in Canada, or nongovernmental, such as nonprofit insurance funds in Germany. At the same time, reforms being undertaken by these national health insurance systems offer evidence of the ways market-based initiatives can address some of the most common problems faced by universal coverage systems.

Even if the United States applies lessons learned from the experience of other nations the country will continue to have a uniquely American system reflective of its cultural preferences—just as every national health care system reflects the cultural, political, and economic systems of the country in which it is found.

Many people gave generously of their time and expertise to assist me in this endeavor. Dr. Sylvester Schieber, vice president of Watson Wyatt and director of Watson Wyatt's Research and Information Center, gave me the freedom and support to complete the third edition of this book. Watson Wyatt's director of legislative affairs, Marjorie Kulash, graciously reviewed numerous drafts. Watson Wyatt consultants who were kind enough to review and comment on my work include global health care practice director Richard Ostuw and consultants Roland McDevitt, Mary Ellen Mullholand, and Mark White. Other Watson Wyatt consultants around the world offered their expertise as well, including Jim Norton, head of the Canadian health care consulting practice; Dr. Chris Brown with the U.K. health care consulting practice; and Ton Pouwels in Amsterdam. Susanne Jungblut and Manuela Walkmann of the Munich office provided excellent information and feedback. Janice Sipus and Peter Miodonski of Watson

Wyatt's Canadian Research and Information Center provided valuable research materials, as did Lisa Loyo of Watson's U.S. Research and Information Center. I am extremely grateful to Kazuhito Ihara, director of the Health and Welfare Department of the Japan External Trade Organization in New York, for his kind assistance with the myriad details of the Japanese health care system. I would also like to thank Debbie Hardin, whose excellent editing skills make this book a more polished product.

The list would not be complete without acknowledging the assistance of my husband Ian, whose loving support and confidence in me have been unwavering.

CHAPTER 1

Health Care:
An International Perspective

A wide array of health care reform initiatives was launched during the decade of the 1990s. Efforts to restructure health care systems became so widespread over the past decade that they assumed the proportions of a "worldwide epidemic" (Klein 1995). These reform efforts were propelled to a large degree by the overriding aim of containing health care cost increases, but they were also driven by the need to increase efficiency while maintaining equity and improving quality. Thus the challenges currently facing the American health care system are not unique; health care systems around the world are struggling to cope with the pressures of rising costs, aging populations, and decisions about how to allocate and pay for seemingly limitless advances in high-technology medical procedures.

The ways in which various nations respond to these shared challenges range from the "Big Bang" approach (Klein 1995) taken by the United Kingdom—which is seeking to remake the centrally run, tightly budgeted National Health Service by embracing such relatively radical market-style concepts as the separation of health care purchasers from providers—to the more gradual incremental reforms implemented in the 1990s in Germany and the Netherlands. Falling somewhere in between has been the market-driven shift in the U.S. health care system from traditional unmanaged fee-for-service arrangements to various forms of managed care.

The search for solutions to shared health care challenges—likened by some to the search for the Holy Grail (Maynard and Hutton, cited in Hsiao 1992)—has been undertaken by nations that have markedly different approaches to the finance, organization, and delivery of health care services. Their differing approaches to both health care and its reforms are shaped by the particular political, economic, cultural, and historical environment of which the health system is a part.

Health care reform would certainly be a far easier task if nations could simply import a one-size-fits-all model to address their shared concerns. It is precisely the important differences rooted in cultural, social, and political factors that make full-scale importation of one nation's

1

health care system impossible, as noted Canadian health economist Robert Evans pointed out:

> Nations do not borrow other nations' institutions. The Canadian system may be "better" than the American.... Even if it is better, I am not trying to sell it to you. You cannot have it. It would not "fit" because you do not see the world, or the individual, or the state, as we do.... *The point is that by examining other people's experience you can extend your range of perceptions of what is possible.* [emphasis added] (Evans 1986, 26)

Thus rather than trying to duplicate another nation's health care system, health care policy makers on the front lines of reform efforts have looked to specific features of other systems that could be shaped and refined for use in their own systems. In so doing, nations have the opportunity to "understand better the key factors that affect one's own health care system" (Hsiao 1992). Viewing the U.S. health care system through the wide-angle lens of an international perspective will allow us to do just that. Indeed, this study aims to extend the reader's range of perceptions of what is possible by providing in-depth analyses of the health care systems of six industrialized nations that have at their disposal a complex array of mechanisms to finance, organize, and deliver health care services to their populations.

HEALTH CARE PARADIGMS

The six nations in this study can be grouped according to the following roughly drawn models:

1. *national health service model* (also known as the Beveridge model), characterized by universal coverage, general tax-based financing, and national ownership and/or control of the factors of production;
2. *social insurance model* (also known as the Bismarck model), characterized by compulsory universal coverage generally within the framework of Social Security and financed by employer and individual contributions through nonprofit insurance funds, and public and/or private ownership of factors of production; and
3. *private insurance model,* characterized by employment-based or individual purchase of private health insurance coverage financed by individual and/or employer contributions and mainly private ownership of the factors of production (OECD 1987, 1994).

Though these models provide a good starting point for classifying different systems, they are limited by the fact that no pure version of any of the systems exists. Most health care systems feature a mix of elements; the United States has a predominantly private system, but nearly half of its finances originate in the public sector; government-run programs for the elderly and the disabled (Medicare) and for lower income individuals (Medicaid) provide care to a significant share of the U.S. population. Germany and the Netherlands rely primarily on the social insurance model, yet private insurance covers a portion of the population. In Japan, employers play a large role in financing the compulsory national health system, and private insurance exists side by side with the National Health Service in the United Kingdom.

Not only do few health care systems fit neatly within the parameters of a single model, but there is a constant balancing act between the roles of the public and private sectors in all activities related to the health care system, from controlling costs to allocating resources (Hsiao 1992). Indeed, though the debate over health care reform often turns on what is frequently presented as a pitched battle of state versus the market, it is not as simple as that; as a recent World Health Organization study pointed out: "Rather than a monolithic commitment to one of two abstractions—state or market—[health care systems] confront a range of smaller decisions" (Saltman and Figueras 1997, 40).

HEALTH SERVICES CONTINUUM

A broader approach to classifying health care systems that further contributes to our understanding of how different health systems are organized and financed and the "uneasy equilibrium" (Anderson 1989, 118) that exists between the public and private sectors was devised by Odin Anderson, a leading health policy scholar with extensive experience in cross-national studies. Anderson locates health care systems along a "health services continuum" (Figure 1-1). The boundaries of the continuum are set by the level of centralization of decision making, particularly over funding for such programs as health care. According to Anderson, "The degree to which a state centralizes financing and planning and the relative size of its public sector determine its position in the continuum, as does the extent to which it intervenes in the operations of the economy itself" (Anderson 1989, 21). Anderson places the United Kingdom's health care system at one extreme—the "market-minimized" pole of the continuum—because its National Health Service is completely government-financed and operated. The United States occupies a position at the opposite extreme—the "market-maximized" end of the continuum. Of course, this is not to deny that there is significant government involvement in the U.S. health care system—particularly with the Medicare and Medicaid programs—but compared to other nations health care services in the United States "have been cut loose in an open field in a way that no other country has conceived of or dared to try" (Anderson 1989, 118). And

FIGURE 1-1   The Market-Minimized/Market-Maximized Continuum

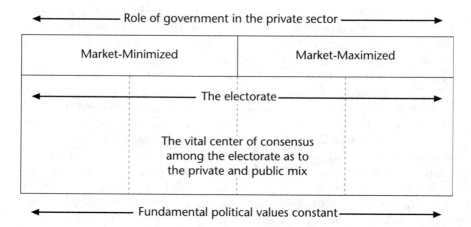

Source: Reprinted from Odin W. Anderson, *Health Care: Can There Be Equity? The United States, Sweden and England*, p. 27. Copyright © 1972 by John Wiley & Sons, Inc. New York. Reprinted by permission of John Wiley & Sons, Inc.

compared to the other nations in this study, the United States has the lowest share of total health expenditures that are publicly funded, whereas the United Kingdom has the highest (Figure 1-2).

Anderson's notion of a continuum underscores the importance of the overall political process and the decision-making roles played by the public and private sectors regarding the development of health care systems. As Anderson noted, "the philosophy of government's counterbalancing private-sector interest groups affects the structure, financing and equity of the health services" (Anderson 1989, 8).

CONVERGENCE AMONG HEALTH SYSTEMS

Through the application of similar health care reform strategies, health care systems have gradually evolved along converging tracks. These efforts represent a search for a compromise position that preserves the best elements of existing systems while selectively adapting processes and techniques that have been successful in other health care systems in addressing shared concerns (Kirkman-Liff 1989).

For example, as noted previously, the U.K. National Health Service, one of the bookends of the continuum, has experimented with market concepts, and likewise the social insurance systems of Germany and the

FIGURE 1-2   Public and Private Financing as a Share of Total Health Expenditures, 1997 (selected countries)

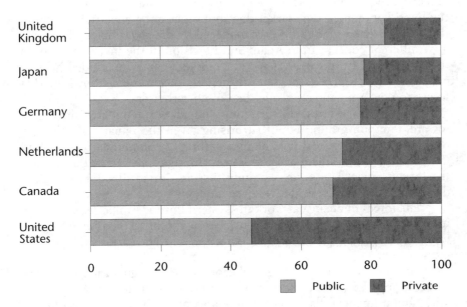

Source: OECD Health Data 98: A Comparative Analysis of 29 Countries. Paris: OECD/CREDES.

Netherlands are looking at how to infuse competition into health systems that are regulated by the government. In the United States, following the rejection of a major broadening of the government's role in the health care sector, the debate now focuses on whether some degree of government regulation is needed as a counterweight to the predominantly competitive free-market principles guiding its health care system.

The common ground on which several health systems are converging is a blend of the free market and government regulation known alternately as the *managed, quasi,* or *internal market.* This "hybrid approach" (Saltman and Figueras 1997) is a close cousin to Stanford University professor Alain Enthoven's managed competition concepts, which combine managed care and market competition and were part of the U.S. health care reform debate in the early 1990s. Now managed markets are a very popular reform prescription and have become one of the American health care sector's major exports (Light 1997).

The introduction of market-style reform elements within regulated systems represents a sea change in terms of how the market is viewed; no longer seen in stark good or bad terms, the market is viewed as a policy tool to be used by government to enhance the efficiency of the health care sector. The market has become "less an antagonist and more . . . an integral and driving force in social policy" (Scheil-Adlung 1998, 104). Within the hybrid approach, the market does not replace the government within the health care system; rather it is managed by the government. Thus it is a far different concept from Adam Smith's vision of the invisible hand; in the context of health care systems, the market's hands are guided by government regulation. At the same time, the government allows market forces to play a much larger role than in an earlier era.

That the continuum is shrinking and that systems are converging toward common ground is not surprising given the remarkable changes occurring around the world. The dismantling of communist regimes and the introduction of free-market practices throughout Eastern Europe and the former Soviet Union are certainly the most vivid illustrations of the dramatic changes that have swept the globe this decade.

The forces of change at work in Western Europe can be seen not only in the reunification of Germany but also in the fifteen-nation European Union's ambitious plan to create a single European market with a common currency.[1]

The emergence of a truly global economy is changing the rules of the game: Money flows around the world without regard to national boundaries, and a financial flashpoint in one area of the world is by no means contained as an isolated event, as born out recently by the way in which financial turmoil in emerging markets in Asia quickly sent shockwaves throughout Europe and the United States.

The hybrid approach—in a sense health care reform's "third way" between a fully competitive market and complete government control—is not unlike developments in the political arena as evidenced by the emergence of such centrist leaders as Bill Clinton in the United States, Tony Blair in the United Kingdom, and Gerhard Schroder in Germany.

The emergence of a more interdependent world, fueled by rapid advances in communications and information technology, has important implications for the health care systems of industrialized countries. Many nations, for example, are realizing the potential benefits that could be enjoyed from working together on approaches to such shared health-related problems as Acquired Immune Deficiency Syndrome (AIDS), cancer, drug addiction, and aging populations (Davis 1990). At the same time, nations are reminded that in a world of free capital and trade flows, corporate investment can shift to nations whose health benefits costs do not impose too heavy a financial burden on employers—further fueling

---

[1] Though there are currently fifteen member nations of the European Union (EU), only eleven will be part of the European Monetary Union (EMU).

the shared search for strategies that control costs and improve efficiency in the health care system.

LIMITS TO CONVERGENCE

The convergence of health care systems seems to be consistent with, and a reflection of, the dramatic tide of change sweeping the world. This convergence is not without its limits, however. Existing differences between health care systems will not disappear, just as a truly borderless world will probably never emerge.

Perhaps the most striking difference separating the U.S. health care system from those of other nations is the philosophical underpinnings of social programs in the United States. The United States places greater emphasis on individual responsibility, free choice, and pluralism, whereas other industrialized nations focus on preserving equitable access to health care for the entire population. The greater involvement of the government in health care financing and delivery in other nations is a reflection of differing philosophical beliefs and social priorities; these differences color perceptions of other systems. As health economist Uwe Reinhardt noted,

> American critics of European health care frequently decry it as two-class medicine—so-called socialized medicine for the poor and private medicine for the rich. Conversely, European critics of American health care frequently depict it as leaning toward Social Darwinism. (Reinhardt 1990, 110)

Even nations such as the United Kingdom and the Netherlands that have recently introduced market-style reforms within their regulated health care systems have opted to retain the tax-based financing structure and commitment to universal coverage. Moreover, the United Kingdom has recently taken several steps back from the market, and the Netherlands has spent a decade attempting to get the right balance of competition and regulation. Thus even reformed health care systems will keep their own trademark characteristics because health care systems are, above all, reflections of the society in which they have evolved: In the final analysis, like politics, all health care is local.

PARAMETERS OF THE STUDY

The shrinking-continuum/limited-convergence theory serves as the framework for this book. The nations whose health care systems are described are situated along various points of the continuum, yet as democracies they have a common basis of public policy formulation that allows various interest groups to participate. Successfully balancing these various interests is critical to health care reform efforts in all nations.

In an attempt to examine health care from a truly global perspective—in geographical, cultural, political, and economic terms—examples are drawn from North America (the United States and Canada), Asia (Japan), and Europe (Germany, the Netherlands, and the United Kingdom). These systems were selected for analyses because they serve as interesting subjects of comparison with the United States, either because of differences or similarities (see Appendix). Indeed, although Americans may feel closer in terms of common heritage and culture to Canada or the United Kingdom, the United States may have more to learn from the public–private mix of the health care systems in Germany and Japan than from the high level of government involvement characteristic of the Canadian and British health systems (Henke 1990; Iglehart 1989; Jonsson 1990).

This book is not designed to compare and contrast different systems in an effort to determine which system is the best, because there is no best system or right or wrong system—no gold standard exists. The imperfectability of health systems and the limits to what they can accomplish was captured rather cleverly by Norwegian Minister of Health Werner Christie: "Some people might even say that the whole health care system is futile, as the average death rate is still 100 percent" (OECD 1996).

Health care reform ideally should involve gradual rather than radical change; the goal really should be to "identify and design politically feasible incremental changes . . . that have a reasonably good chance of making things better" (Enthoven 1990, 58). As the health care systems of industrialized countries evolve and converge, each country stands to gain from the experience of others going through similar changes. This study is intended to provide a sound basis for understanding how other industrialized nations organize and finance their health care systems, and thereby enhance awareness of the range of what is possible.

CHAPTER 2

Managing the
U.S. Health Care System

This tour through international health care systems begins at the market-maximized pole of Anderson's continuum. The United States has a mixture of public and private programs and plans that provide health insurance coverage and services to various segments—but not all—of the population. The U.S. health care system is often heralded as the best in the world, particularly because it provides the most advanced medical care. Though it has much to commend it, serious challenges in the form of cost, access, and quality of care continue to weigh on the system.

This chapter provides an overview of the rapidly changing U.S. health care system and opens with a description of the various programs that provide insurance coverage to the majority of the U.S. population. The second section of the chapter takes a look back in time to examine the forces that led to the proposed Clinton administration health care reform plan. The third section examines the dramatic shift from traditional unlimited fee-for-service indemnity insurance to managed care and the impact of this shift on health care costs. The chapter closes with a discussion of what changes may be in store for the U.S. health care system.

A SYSTEM IN CONSTANT FLUX

Though the U.S. health care system has undergone profound changes over the past three decades, the one constant throughout this period has been a sense, real or perceived, of a crisis in the American health care system. At a 1969 press conference President Richard Nixon spoke of a "massive crisis" in health care, and warned that "unless action is taken in the next two to three years . . . we will have a breakdown in our medical system" (Starr 1982, 381). A 1970 survey found three out of four Americans agreed that the U.S. health care system was in crisis (Starr 1982). Dire proclamations of crisis and turmoil in the health care arena in the 1980s helped propel Bill Clinton into the White House in 1992 and were at the heart of the formulation of his far-reaching plan to dramatically reform the U.S. health care system.

The U.S. health care system—one seventh of the U.S. economy—is currently at the tail end of a decade of fundamental restructuring driven by market-based competition with large employers—the major health care bill payers—essentially in the driver's seat. The traditional fee-for-service, largely unrestricted, health care plans that provided the dominant form of coverage in the United States for more than half a century have been re-placed by a wide range of plans broadly described as those that manage care.[1]

The U.S. health care system has never been easy to explain—witness the terms most commonly used to describe it: complex, uncoordinated, loosely structured, fragmented, nondesigned—and even harder to com-prehend.[2] The intensity and velocity of the changes affecting the system over the past decade make this task even more daunting, particularly be-cause the current situation is likely to be a mere pit stop en route to a fu-ture reconfiguration of the U.S. health care system.

No health care system exists in a vacuum; rather it is a reflection of the particular cultural, political, and economic factors of the society of which it is a part, and it is important to point out that the United States differs from the other nations studied in several important ways. For ex-ample, the U.S. population is generally more heterogeneous than that of other nations examined in this study; the American public has a more pro-found distrust of government coupled with a stronger aversion to taxes; and the United States has a long history of preferring the private sector over the public sector in terms of the delivery and management of health care services and costs.

As subsequent chapters will show, other nations rely on governmen-tally imposed measures such as uniform fee schedules, global budgets, or expenditure caps on specific health sectors to control costs. The U.S. Medicare program uses the prospective payment system (PPS) to set prices and per capita payments to hospitals and the resource-based relative value scale (RBRVS) and volume performance standards (VPS) to set reimburse-ment rates for physicians and limits on the volume of services provided. Private sector health plans use various tools of managed care, such as lim-ited choice of providers, selective contracting, gatekeepers, and utilization

---

[1] It is important to note that fee-for-service has not disappeared as many types of managed care plans pay for services on a *discounted* fee-for-service basis.

[2] Several excellent discussions of the U.S. health care system include Joseph White (1995), *Competing Solutions: American Health Care Proposals and International Experience;* John Iglehart's series (1992a, 1992b, 1992c, 1992d, 1993a, 1993b, 1994a, 1994b, 1994c, 1995a, 1995b, 1996, 1997a, 1997b) on the American health care system in the *New England Journal of Medicine,* vari-ous issues 1992–present; and OECD, *The Reform of Health Care in Seventeen OECD Countries.*

FIGURE 2-1   Health Care Expenditures, 1970–1997 (in percentages of GDP)

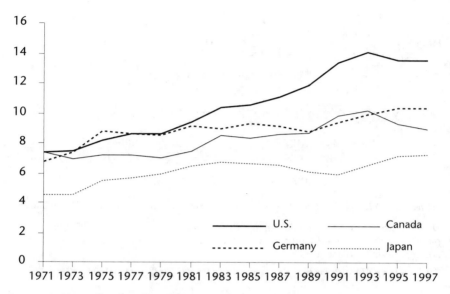

Source: OECD Health Data 98: A Comparative Analysis of 29 Countries. Paris: OECD/CREDES.

control to manage costs. These methods have successfully slowed the rate of increase in U.S. health care spending over the past several years.

Despite managed care's cost control successes, however, health care spending consumes nearly 14 percent of the U.S. Gross Domestic Product (GDP),[3] far more than in any other industrialized nation (Figure 2–1). U.S. per capita health care spending exceeds that of the next most expensive systems in this study, namely Germany and Canada, by a wide margin (Figure 2–2).

The financing side of the $1.1 trillion the United States spent on health care in 1997 was split between public (46 percent) and private (54 percent) sources.[4] Private health insurance represented nearly one-third of all health care funds. On the expenditure side, the hospital sector accounted for more than one-third of all expenditures, and physicians' services came in second at one-fifth of all expenditures (Table 2–1).

---

[3] National health expenditures (NHE) as a percentage of GDP measures the share of national resources devoted to health care. GDP, a commonly used measure of economic growth, represents the total market value of all goods and services produced *domestically.* GDP differs from the Gross National Product (GNP), which also includes the value of goods and services produced by companies and citizens abroad.

[4] The public share of total health expenditures has risen from 40 percent in 1990 to 46 percent in 1998.

FIGURE 2-2   Per Capita Spending on Health Care, 1997 (in $U.S.)

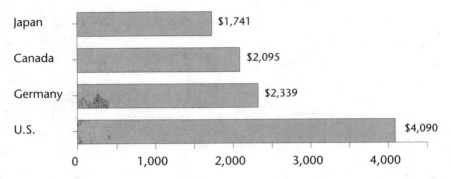

Source: OECD Health Data 98: A Comparative Analysis of 29 Countries. Paris: OECD/CREDES.

Note: Per capita spending is adjusted for purchasing power parities (PPPs). PPPs express the rate at which one currency should be converted to another to purchase the same set of goods and services in both countries.

Of the more than 5,000 community hospitals[5] in the United States, 15 percent are for-profit investor-owned institutions, and 26 percent are owned by state and local governments. The large majority—59 percent—of community hospitals are owned by nongovernmental not-for-profit organizations (Stevens 1998). These not-for-profit hospitals accounted for more than 70 percent of all expenses, personnel, births, and outpatient visits in 1996.

The reorganization of the U.S. health care system over the past decade has led to a significant change in the physician landscape. Whereas solo practitioners and small partnerships were once the norm, increasing numbers of physicians are now part of large group practices. The share of physicians in solo practice dropped from 41 percent in 1983 to 29 percent in 1994. According to the American Medical Association, the number of group practices rose from 17,000 in 1991 to 20,000 in 1995, with the average number of physicians per practice increasing from 6.6 to 10.5 over that time period (Kletke, Emmons, and Gillis 1996). Whereas fewer than one quarter of all doctors worked for someone else—in other words, were not self-employed—in 1983, 43 percent of physicians are now employees of HMOs, hospitals, or physician practice management firms (Stolberg 1998).

---

[5] Community hospitals are defined as all nonfederal short-term general and other special hospitals whose facilities and services are open to the public.

TABLE 2–1   U.S. Health Care Dollars: Where They Came From, Where They Went, 1997

Revenues by major payer	As percentage of total health care payments	Health care expenditures by major category	As percentage of total health care expenditures
Private health insurance	31.9	Hospitals	34.0
Medicare	19.6	Physicians	19.9
Out-of-pocket	17.2	Nursing homes	7.6
Medicaid	14.6	Prescription drugs	7.2
Other government	12.2	Administration	4.6
Other private	4.6	Other	26.7

Source: Health Care Financing Administration; "National Health Expenditures 1997: The Nation's Health Dollar 1997," at www.hcfa.gov/stats/nhe.

HEALTH INSURANCE COVERAGE IN THE UNITED STATES

In contrast to a comprehensive system of national health insurance or a national health service that exists in other nations, the majority of the U.S. population receives health insurance coverage through a patchwork of public and private programs with varying levels of benefits.

PUBLIC PROGRAMS

The two major publicly funded health care programs—Medicare and Medicaid—date back to 1965. Together these programs account for one-third of all U.S. health care spending and provide coverage to approximately 80 million Americans. These two programs represent the U.S. version of mandatory health insurance, although coverage is limited to the elderly, the disabled, and some segments of the low-income population.

Medicare is the single largest payer of health care services in the predominantly private U.S. health care system; it was responsible for one-fifth of total U.S. health care spending in 1997 for nearly 40 million aged and disabled beneficiaries. Medicare provides health care services to individuals aged 65 and older (as well as to disabled individuals and those with permanent kidney failure). It is a two-part program: Part A covers inpatient hospital care as well as limited nursing home care, home health care visits, and hospice care, and is financed through the hospital insurance (HI) payroll tax,[6] and individual cost-sharing in the form of deductibles

---

[6] Employers and employees pay equal shares of the payroll tax, which amounts to 2.9 percent of the employee's wages.

and coinsurance. Medicare Part B provides partial payments for physician services, outpatient hospital services, rural health clinic office visits, and related physician supplies. It is financed through general tax revenues and individual premiums (Fronstin and Copeland 1997).

Given that Part A of the Medicare program is financed by payroll taxes, demographics is wreaking havoc on the program's finances: As the population ages, the number of people paying into the system will decline relative to the number drawing benefits. Measures to bolster the system's finances include options such as raising the eligibility age for full benefits from 65 to 67; imposing means-testing on parts of the program; and imposing copayments for certain services. Though such measures have not yet been enacted, they will likely be reconsidered in the near future (Fronstin and Copeland 1997).

The Medicaid program is jointly financed by federal and state governments,[7] and provides coverage for certain categories of low-income people, including children, elderly people, blind people, or disabled people, as well as people who receive federal income assistance. Total spending for 41 million Medicaid beneficiaries approached $160 billion in 1997. No distinct program to provide coverage for long-term care exists in the United States. The Medicaid program covered nearly one-third and Medicare an additional one quarter of the total $92 billion spent on nursing home and related services in 1995 (U.S. GAO 1998a).

Other publicly funded health care programs include federal, state, and local government programs. The Federal Employees Health Benefit Plan (FEHBP) provides health insurance coverage to 9 million employees of the federal government and their dependents, and employees of state and local governments are covered through state-level programs such as the California Public Employee Retirement System (CalPERS), which provides health insurance for more than 1 million enrollees. Finally, CHAMPUS (Civilian Health and Medical Program of the Uniformed Services) and CHAMPVA (Civilian Health and Medical Program of the Veteran's Administration) programs provide coverage for dependents of active duty and retired members of the uniformed services.

THE PRIVATE HEALTH INSURANCE SECTOR

The bulk of the U.S. population is covered by private health insurance through the workplace. More than 60 percent of the population is covered through group health plans tied to employment—either their own em-

---

[7] The federal share ranges from 50 to 83 percent of expenditures, depending on the state's per capita income level. In 1997 total Medicaid expenditures were roughly 60 percent federal to 40 percent state.

FIGURE 2-3   Health Insurance Coverage, 1997 (as percentage of the population)

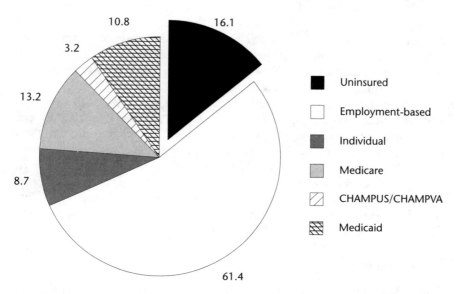

Source: U.S. Department of Commerce, Economics and Statistics Administration, Census Bureau, *Current Population Reports, Health Insurance Coverage: 1997* (September 1998).

Note: Total exceeds 100 percent because of multiple sources of health insurance coverage.

ployment or through a family member.[8] A much smaller group purchases private insurance on their own (Figure 2–3). Until the early 1990s traditional indemnity fee-for-service health insurance plans were the dominant form of employment-based coverage. As discussed in more detail later in the chapter, a wide range of managed care arrangements has taken the place of such plans, which currently represent fewer than 15 percent of all employment-sponsored health coverage.

American businesses fell into the role of predominant health insurance sponsor—a role assumed primarily by the government in most nations—to a certain degree by accident; during the 1940s a wartime freeze on wages prevented employers from competing for scarce workers on the basis of higher salaries. The freeze did not apply to employer contributions to employee health insurance coverage, however, and employers offered attractive health benefit packages to entice workers (Fuchs 1994; Starr 1982). Although employers sponsor health insurance plans for their

---

[8] Employers provide coverage to their active as well as retired employees. In 1996, for example, approximately one-third of individuals aged 65 and older had employment-based coverage—mainly as a supplement to coverage under the Medicare program (Fronstin 1998).

employees on a voluntary basis, government tax incentives have encouraged businesses to provide benefits because employer-sponsored health insurance premiums are treated as a tax-deduction for the employer but are not included in an employee's taxable income. The voluntary nature of the U.S. system provides an avenue of competitive advantage for employers—typically large employers—that can afford to offer rich benefit packages to entice the highest quality workers to join their firms.

Other nations studied here have employment-based health insurance systems (Germany and Japan, for instance), but these systems feature employer mandates—which are notably absent in the U.S. system. Only one U.S. state, Hawaii, requires employers to provide insurance for their employees (Graig 1993).[9] President Clinton's proposed 1993 health care reform plan featured a mandate on employers to purchase health insurance for their employees; the mandate—and accompanying government bureaucracy needed to administer and enforce it—was widely viewed as one of the major reasons for the plan's failure.

THE UNINSURED

The U.S. system's disjointed nature—a series of unconnected programs covering various groups in the population—creates gaps through which a significant share of the population falls. In 1997 more than 16 percent of the U.S. population[10] was without health insurance coverage—though not necessarily access to care—at any one time. This "paradox of excess and deprivation" (Enthoven and Kronick 1989, 29), with the United States spending more than $1 trillion on health care in 1997 while 43 million individuals go without coverage, sets the private voluntary insurance-based United States apart from other nations in this study.

Many of those without insurance pay for health care services directly, and others receive care through public clinics and hospitals and state and local health programs. Others receive charity[11] or uncompensated care

---

[9] Hawaii's 1974 Prepaid Health Care Act requires employers to provide the state-mandated minimum benefits package to all employees working at least 20 hours per week. The act took effect before the enactment of the federal Employee Retirement Income Security Act (ERISA) of 1974, which prevents additional states from enacting similar mandates. ERISA generally supersedes or preempts all state laws otherwise applicable to pension and welfare plans covered by ERISA, with the exception of state laws regulating insurance, banking, and securities. In 1983 Hawaii was granted a limited exemption from ERISA's preemption clause; this preserved the Hawaii statute as of 1974, but not any subsequent amendments to the law (EBRI 1995).

[10] The uninsured are often expressed as a percentage of the nonelderly population (see Figure 2–12) because all those age 65 and older are covered by the Medicare program. In 1997 18.3 percent of the *nonelderly* population was uninsured.

[11] The American Medical Association estimated that physicians provide $3 billion worth of free services and nearly $4 billion of reduced-fee services annually (OECD 1994). The American Hospital Association estimated that hospitals provided more than $13 billion in uncompensated care in 1991 (Fronstin 1997). Under Medicaid's Disproportionate Share Hospital payments program, hospitals are compensated for serving a disproportionate share of low-income patients.

from private providers, the cost of which is shifted to other health care payers who pay more than the full cost of the health care they receive to cover the cost of care for the uninsured. Such uncompensated care is a critical safety valve in a system without universal coverage (Smith 1997). Under the traditional system of fee-for-service payments there was more wiggle room for such cost-shifting, but the current dominance of managed care's cost-saving techniques sharply curtails providers' ability to pass along these costs to other payers (Aaron 1996a).

The large and growing uninsured population in the United States is a direct byproduct of U.S. inability to come to agreement over whether health care is a right to which all are entitled regardless of income level or a private consumer good available only to those who can afford to purchase it or receive it as a benefit of employment (Reinhardt 1996a 1997). Though the latter position was reaffirmed by the demise of the Clinton health care reform plan, it would be shortsighted to consider that the end of the story. The issue of universal coverage surfaces at regular intervals; the United States has started down the road to national health insurance (or at least looked at the maps and plotted a trip) numerous times over the course of the past century (Aaron 1996a; Iglehart 1992d; Marmor 1993; Skocpol 1995; Starr 1982). Our long-running ping-pong match with national health insurance ensures that health care reform, particularly the issues of expanding and guaranteeing access to the entire population, will continue to command a central position on the U.S. public policy agenda.

BACK TO THE FUTURE

A brief look back enables us to better understand the current state of U.S. health care and the pressures that have driven dramatic changes in the system over the past decade. The 1980s witnessed a tremendous increase in the cost of health care. At that time the U.S. health care system was dominated by traditional indemnity insurance, fee-for-service payment arrangements to doctors who were mainly in solo or small group practices, free choice of doctor and hospital, and a third-party intermediary that shielded those receiving care from the true cost of services. The forces of cost-increasing incentives built into the fee-for-service system and the cost-unconsciousness of insured patients combined to create an explosive mixture of runaway costs (Enthoven 1993). Unlike other nations that relied on various governmental levers to control costs, no such central control over health care costs existed, and those paying the bills had no meaningful leverage over those providing the services (Aaron 1996a).

By the mid-1980s U.S. companies, the major payers of the health care tab (for employee health insurance premiums, the employer portion of

FIGURE 2-4   Private Business Health Expenditures, 1980–1990 (in $ billions)

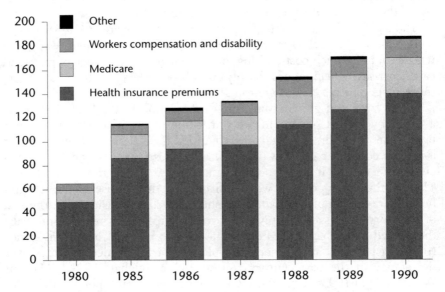

Source: Health Care Financing Administration, Office of National Health Statistics, quoted in Levit and Cowan "Business, households, and governments: Health care costs, 1990." *Health Care Financing Review* 13, no. 2.

Medicare taxes, and the medical portion of workers' compensation) (Figure 2–4) cried out for relief. Many U.S. companies complained that high health care costs put them at a competitive disadvantage with regard to foreign competitors in countries with nationalized health care systems. General Motors, the largest single private U.S. health care purchaser, for instance, frequently pointed out that it spent more on health care for its employees—GM's 1988 health care bill topped the $3 billion mark—than it did for the steel it used to make automobiles (Freudenheim 1989a, 1989b, 1989c).[12]

Most large companies had already taken some steps to become more directly involved in overseeing employee health care costs. Most notably they had set up self-insured plans, which essentially meant that rather than paying premiums to insurance companies in advance, the employer pays for employee health claims as they occur. In addition to affording the employer savings in premiums paid to insurance companies and tighter control over cash flow, a significant benefit of self-insurance was the pro-

---

[12] By 1996 the big three car manufacturers (GM, Ford, and Chrysler) combined spent nearly $7 billion on health care for their employees (Freudenheim 1998a).

tection from differing state regulations accorded such plans by the 1974 Employee Retirement Income Security Act (ERISA). Under ERISA, self-insured plans are not subject to state insurance premium taxes and are exempt from state-mandated benefit laws.

Larger employers are far more likely to self-insure their health benefits plans than smaller employers, who have a more difficult time finding ways to control costs and are hit particularly hard by skyrocketing costs. They pay higher health premiums than larger companies, and are unable to spread either risk or costs as widely as large companies (Levit and Cowan 1991; O'Keefe 1992). Many smaller employers were forced to drop their plans altogether, contributing to the rising pool of uninsured and increasing the strain on other companies, which ended up covering those uninsured individuals as dependents of their workers.

The costs of retiree health care also featured prominently in the debate. Given the aging of the U.S. work force, the provision of health care coverage for individuals who retire before the age of 65 and are therefore not yet eligible for coverage under the Medicare program is a significant concern. The escalating cost of health care forced many companies to drop or seriously curtail the extent of health care benefits provided to retirees. Accounting standards issued by the Financial Accounting Standards Board (FASB)[13] requiring companies to carry the financial liability for postretirement medical care benefits on their balance sheets intensified corporate America's call for relief from rising health care costs.

Whereas in 1980 few employers viewed health care costs as a major problem, by the end of the decade, as the annual rate of inflation in health insurance premiums approached 20 percent, that was no longer the prevailing view (Bodenhimer and Sullivan 1998). A 1990 survey of almost 2,000 senior executives across a broad range of industries revealed that nearly two-thirds of respondents believed health benefits costs to be the leading issue companies faced at that time (Wyatt Company 1990). Some business executives even suggested that the United States might take the unusual step of supporting a closer look at a Canadian-style system of national health insurance (Freudenheim 1989b).

Employees were faced with a tradeoff between the continuation of health insurance benefits and hoped-for wage increases. Because such benefits as health insurance are exempt from taxes, many workers prefer such tax-free noncash compensation over taxable wage increases (Fuchs 1994). Disputes over health benefits were a continuing flashpoint of industrial relations as workers fought not only to preserve existing benefits but to cur-

---

[13] Though Financial Accounting Standard (FAS) 106 took effect for fiscal years beginning after December 15, 1992, companies had already begun to prepare for the accounting standard by the late 1980s.

tail employers' attempts to shift larger portions of health care costs to them (Carnevale 1989; Crenshaw 1989). According to the Bureau of Labor Statistics, the average monthly premium contribution paid by full-time employees in large firms (100 or more employees), for example, increased nearly 25 percent from 1980 to 1991.

Access to health care continued to be a problem as the numbers of uninsured approached 35 million by the end of the 1980s. A large share of the uninsured were working adults, particularly those in small companies (25 or fewer employees), and in firms with primarily low-wage workers. Insecurity grew among working Americans—even those with insurance—who feared that they might one day be without health insurance.

A 1990 poll found that 90 percent of Americans surveyed believed that the U.S. health care system required fundamental change or a complete rebuilding (Blendon, Leitman, Morrison, and Donelan 1990). Other polls at that time revealed that support for national health insurance was at its highest level since the 1950s (Blendon, Bodie, and Benson 1995).

HEALTH CARE REFORM TAKES CENTER STAGE

It was against this backdrop that Bill Clinton was elected president in 1992, and he promised to make the troubled U.S. health care system a top domestic priority. He placed First Lady Hillary Rodham Clinton in charge of the health care reform effort.

The Clinton plan[14] was modeled on an approach known as *managed competition*. This strategy, developed by Stanford University economist Alain Enthoven, physician Paul Ellwood, and others, aimed to achieve the twin goals of cost control and improved efficiency of the health care system by encouraging health plans to compete on the basis of cost and quality. This competition would not be unfettered, however. Large purchasing cooperatives dubbed "sponsors" would "manage" the competition in their role as intermediaries between health plans and individuals.[15]

The president's highly complex reform plan, known as the Health Security Act, was unveiled in September 1993. The proposed health plan

---

[14] Volumes have been written on the Clinton plan's birth, short life, and demise. A very small sampling includes Joseph White (1995) *Competing Solutions;* Victor Fuchs (1994b), "The Clinton Plan: A Researcher Examines Reform"; Reinhardt (1994), "The Clinton Plan: A Salute to American Pluralism"; John Iglehart (1993b), "The Labyrinth of Congress" Daniel Yankelovich (1995), "The Debate that Wasn't: The Public and the Clinton Plan"; Theda Skocpol (1995), "The Rise and Resounding Demise of the Clinton Plan."

[15] Shades of Enthoven's unique blend of competition and regulation were evident in the president's proposal, even though Enthoven would ultimately argue that the Clinton plan's all too heavy reliance on an expanded role for federal and state governments strayed too far from managed competition's core concepts to be worthy of the name (Enthoven and Singer 1994).

guaranteed universal coverage through a mandate on employers to pay the bulk of the premium cost of a standard benefits package for their employees, with subsidies provided for smaller companies, low-wage workers, early retirees, and the unemployed. All Americans would obtain insurance by joining either a state-run regional alliance or, if they were employees of a large company, a corporate purchasing alliance.

In his January 1994 State of the Union address, President Clinton drew a line in the sand with the following challenge to Congress: "If you send me legislation that does not guarantee every American private health insurance that can never be taken away, you will force me to take this pen, veto the legislation, and we'll come right back here and start all over again" (reported in Iglehart July 1994a). This was the Clinton health care version of Patrick Henry's famous call for liberty: "Give me universal coverage or give me death." Unfortunately for the president, the latter option was most publicly bestowed on his reform plan by year's end.

Dubbed by many experts as "doomed from the start" (Iglehart 1998), the president's plan sank under the weight of numerous factors. Most important, powerful forces arrayed themselves against the plan. The insurance and health care industries the plan sought to regulate; employers of all sizes that balked at mandated coverage; and a good portion of the public, which struggled to understand the highly complicated plan—all were vocal opponents.

The plan's reliance on an expanded governmental regulatory apparatus collided with strong public cynicism about allowing the government such a large role in managing one-seventh of the U.S. economy. Opponents of the plan made the comparison to another government-run bureaucracy, pointing out that "if you like the U.S. Postal Service, you'll love the Clinton health plan." Indeed, opponents used the heavy role of government to pin the opprobrium of socialized medicine on the plan, ensuring it would never gain widespread support in a nation that had a marked preference for private-sector solutions to health care problems (Blendon et al. 1995; Ginzberg 1998; Iglehart 1994b, 1998; Skocpol 1995). If these factors were not enough, the plan was further handicapped by having to share congressional attention with a panoply of competing proposals ranging from several other managed competition-type reform plans to those based on a Canadian-style single-payer system. In the final analysis, although there was a significant degree of dissatisfaction with the U.S. health care system, there was woefully limited consensus on an appropriate alternative.

The battle over health care reform essentially came down to a face-off between the heavy hand of government versus the invisible hand of the market. Invisible won, hands down, as market competition muscled government regulation out of the way. The failed Clinton plan did not cause the market-driven reforms that currently characterize the U.S. health care system, because those forces were already at work, but the full-scale rejection of a reformed system featuring an expanded role for government gave a significant push to such ongoing private sector efforts. Indeed, the great irony was that some of the specific health care delivery and financing arrangements of the never-enacted Clinton plan—most notably competing managed care plans—swiftly took hold, and since that point the U.S. health care system has been dramatically transformed.

MANAGED CARE'S TRANSFORMATION
OF THE U.S. HEALTH CARE SYSTEM

The broad range of changes envisioned by the proposed legislation never came to pass, but the U.S. health care system has been transformed nonetheless. After a decade of unrelenting premium increases, employers—the major payers of health care services in the United States—staged what has been described as a "buyers revolt" (Light 1998) and forced significant changes in the way health care is paid for and organized in the United States.

In the wake of this revolt, the health care lexicon has come to feature a bewildering array of acronyms—what one analyst refers to as a "Tower of Babel" of managed care terminology—HMOs, PPOs, POS, and so on. Health care professionals—be they physicians, hospitals, pharmacists, and so on—are now known as *providers*, and patients are referred to as *health care consumers*.

Employers have shifted their employees from traditional unrestricted fee-for-service indemnity health plans into a range of plans that although different in significant aspects aim to control costs and fall under the broad rubric of managed care. The spectrum of managed care arrangements encompasses health maintenance organizations (HMOs)—which essentially married two previously separate functions: the financing side that insurers had taken care of by paying health claims and the delivery side previously dominated by the physicians who determined how and what health care services were provided—as well as less restrictive arrangements such as preferred provider organizations (PPOs), which feature a select panel of providers that contracts with employers to provide health benefits at discounted fees, and hybrid plans such as point-of-service (POS) plans, which feature elements of HMOs and PPOs by allowing members the option to pay more to use out-of-network providers.

Managed care can be viewed in the context of strategies to manage physician practice and thus control costs; as health economist Uwe Reinhardt explained, it is a system of "external control over the clinical decisions of individual patients and their physicians concerning the treatment of given medical conditions" (Reinhardt 1995). Some of the many methods used by health plans to manage care include utilization review; hospital preadmission certification; mandatory second opinion before surgery; the use of primary care physicians as gatekeepers; payment of providers on the basis of capitated payments rather than fee-for-service; and incentives or requirements for patients to use the plan's facilities and doctors.

Managed care, far from being the new kid on the health care block, has been around for nearly half a century in the form of prepaid group practices, dating back to Los Angeles's Ross Loos clinic and the Group Health Association of Washington, D.C., in the 1930s; and Kaiser Permanente, Group Health of Puget Sound, and New York's Health Insurance Plan (HIP) in the 1940s (Iglehart 1992a; Mayer and Mayer 1985; Starr 1982). These nonprofit health plans, essentially closed systems with doctors on salary and a focus on preventive care, were considered radical upstarts at a time when few Americans had health insurance coverage; indeed these plans were viewed by most physicians with disdain similar to that accorded socialized medicine at that time (Kuttner 1998).[16]

In the early 1970s the Nixon administration seized on these prepaid plans as a way to stem health care expenditure growth. Indeed, the administration looked favorably on Kaiser's experience, providing prepaid health care services for 20 to 40 percent less than fee-for-service medicine. The administration adopted the name "health maintenance organization" (HMO) put forth by Paul Ellwood, a Minneapolis physician considered the father of HMOs, for the new health care arrangements that receive fixed payment in advance for each enrollee regardless of how much health care the individual consumed (Starr 1982). HMO enrollees receive comprehensive benefits from a defined network of providers and in general select a primary care physician, or "gatekeeper," who controls access to specialists.

The vehicle for the Nixon administration's "health maintenance strategy" was the 1973 Health Maintenance Organization Act, which featured subsidies to foster the growth of HMOs; the law also set broad coverage standards for federally qualified HMOs. The law's goal was to create 1,700 HMOs to serve 40 million members by 1976. Though actual HMO enrollment only topped 6 million members by that year, the law served as an important catalyst for the burgeoning HMO industry (Iglehart 1992c).

FROM THERE TO HERE

The 1973 HMO legislation laid the critical foundation for the expansion of managed care, yet fee-for-service arrangements continued to dominate

---

[16] Many of these plans are still thriving one-half century after their birth. Group Health of Puget Sound is now the largest health plan in the Northwest, with nearly 700,000 members; Kaiser, for its part, has a nationwide presence and provides services to more than 9 million enrollees (Kuttner 1998).

FIGURE 2-5   Managed Care Ascendent (percentage of insured persons by type of plan)

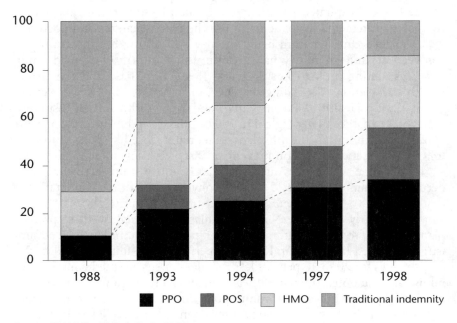

Source: KPMG Health Benefits in 1998.

the health care arena until the mid-1980s. At that point corporate America, driven by the overarching goal of controlling employee health care costs, dove headfirst into managed care and all its manifestations. From the late 1980s throughout the 1990s, traditional unrestricted fee-for-service plans staged an amazing disappearing act, as coverage shrank from more than 70 percent of all privately insured employees in 1988 to 14 percent in 1998 (Figure 2–5). Even the fee-for-service plans that remain now feature elements of managed care (i.e., precertification or utilization review), whereas virtually none did in 1980. Large employers were the pioneers, but small employers hopped on the managed care bandwagon seemingly overnight. In 1993 nearly 80 percent of small employers (those with fewer than 25 employees) offered a conventional fee-for-service plan; in two years this dropped dramatically to 30 percent (Jensen, Morrisey, Gaffney, and Liston 1997). Moreover, the vast majority of federal employees are now in managed care plans of various types.

By 1992 HMO enrollment had finally reached the goal set in the 1973 legislation. HMOs have changed much from the days of the nonprofit plans of the 1940s, however. Only Minnesota requires HMOs to be non-

FIGURE 2-6   HMO and PPO Enrollment, 1990–1996 (in millions of persons)

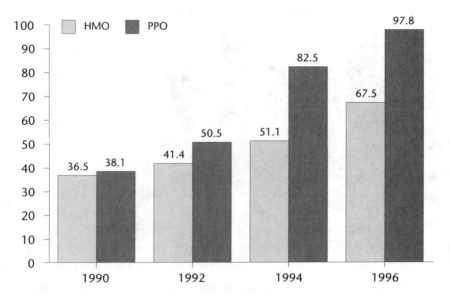

Source: 1995–1996 AAHP HMO and PPO Trends Report. Washington, D.C.: American Association of Health Plans.

profit organizations, and more than 60 percent of all HMO enrollees are in for-profit plans today, up from 12 percent in 1981. For-profit HMOs now represent three quarters of all health plans, up from less than one-fifth in 1981 (Kuttner 1998; Srinivasen, Levitt, and Lundy 1998).

Though HMOs currently provide coverage for 30 percent of insured Americans, enrollment growth has been particularly dramatic among plans such as preferred provider organizations (PPOs) that offer more free-dom in terms of the choice of health care provider. PPOs selectively con-tract with a network of doctors and hospitals to provide services at dis-counted rates, in return for higher patient volume. PPO enrollees have a financial incentive to use the PPO's designated network-affiliated pro-viders; if they choose to go outside the network for care they pay a higher copayment rate. The number of persons enrolled in PPOs nearly tripled between 1990 and 1996 (Figure 2–6). Not only are employees choosing such plans, but employers are increasingly offering them; the largest share of responding companies in Watson Wyatt's 1997–1998 survey report on employee benefits considered their PPO plan to be their primary plan (Figure 2–7).

FIGURE 2-7   Percentage of Employers Offering Plan as Primary Plan, and Percentage Change, 1995–1998

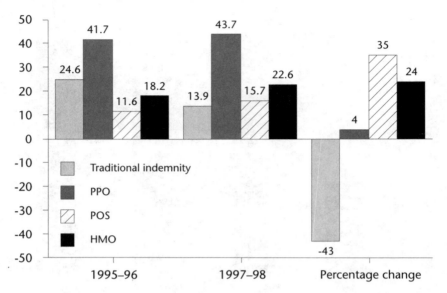

Source: The ECS Survey Report on Employee Benefits 1998/9 (Watson Wyatt Data Service).

Point-of-service plans (POSs) also give members the option of going outside the HMO network for health care services at higher cost to the patient. These plans have become increasingly popular because they offer greater freedom of choice and less restrictions than traditional closed-panel HMOs.

Despite the fact that HMOs and PPOs together now provide care to more than 170 million Americans, the expansive growth of managed care has not been evenly distributed throughout all regions of the United States. Twelve states had fewer than one-tenth of their populations in HMOs in 1996, and only ten states had 30 percent or more of their population in managed care arrangements. Contrast California, for example, home of the original HMOs, with 42 percent of its population enrolled in an HMO—90 percent of all *insured* residents of its state capital Sacramento are in HMOs—with rural states such as Wyoming, North Dakota, and Montana, where well under 5 percent of the population is enrolled in a HMO. Rural areas lack the population density necessary to support integrated health plans and may have physician shortages rather than surpluses (Albert 1998a).

Managed care has also made its way—bolstered by federal and state initiatives—into the Medicare and Medicaid programs. The most common vehicle of managed care coverage for Medicare beneficiaries is through a Medicare HMO. Medicare HMOs entice beneficiaries who lack or have limited employer-sponsored coverage to join by offering lower deductibles and coinsurance rates. In 1997, for example, nearly 70 percent of Medicare HMOs did not charge beneficiaries a monthly premium (AAHP 1998). Medicare HMOs tend to offer a richer benefit package as well, one that may cover services not covered by traditional fee-for-service Medicare such as routine physicals, eye and ear exams, and prescription drugs.

Enrollment in Medicare managed care has tripled since 1989, reaching 6 million—15 percent of all beneficiaries—in 1997. Again, the growth of managed care has been unevenly distributed; 4 states account for more than one-half of all Medicare managed care enrollees. Though experts predict that Medicare managed care enrollment will peak at the 25 to 30 percent of beneficiaries mark, the growth potential is considered to be significant given that one in four Medicare beneficiaries live in areas without an HMO (nearly 20 states do not have an HMO that serves the Medicare population). Managed care will also get a boost under the new Medicare + Choice program created as part of the Balanced Budget Act of 1997. Also known as Medicare Part C, this program expands the range of private plan options available to Medicare beneficiaries to include provider-sponsored organizations, private fee-for-service plans, preferred provider organizations, point-of-service plans, and medical savings accounts.

The Balanced Budget Act limited federal Medicare reimbursement rates, and some HMOs are currently pulling out of certain Medicare managed care markets as they have found these rates to be unacceptably low in the face of rising costs. The withdrawals have affected fewer than 5 percent of all Medicare HMO enrollees. At the same time that plans are pulling out of certain regions where their profit margins are too slim, new plans have applied for acceptance as Medicare HMOs, so the ultimate impact of the pull-outs remains to be seen.

Managed care has made far more significant inroads into the Medicaid program, driven by state efforts to rein in exploding Medicaid expenditures. Enrollment of Medicaid beneficiaries in managed care quadrupled between 1991 and 1996, rising to more than 13 million in 1996. As of 1997 nearly half of all Medicaid beneficiaries were in managed care plans. Continued growth will be bolstered by the provisions of the Balanced Budget Act of 1997 that expand the authority of state Medicaid agencies to enroll beneficiaries in managed care without the previously required federal waiver from the Department of Health and Human Services.

MANAGED CARE'S IMPACT ON PROVIDER PAYMENT

Businesses through their "buyers revolt" provided the spark for the shift from unrestricted fee-for-service health insurance coverage to managed care plans, and it was the fat in the system that has sustained the explosive growth in managed care. The system's excess capacity—low hospital occupancy rates, oversupply of advanced medical technology, and over-supply of specialists—enabled managed care organizations to negotiate discounted prices with health care professionals, which in turn enabled these organizations to charge lower premiums to their enrollees and capture a dominant share of the health care market (Fuchs 1997).

Though discounted fee-for-service remains the dominant payment method, some managed care organizations transfer risk to physicians through a payment method known as *capitation*. Under a capitated system, physicians are paid a fixed amount per month per enrolled member of the plan, rather than a fee for each service provided. In the premanaged care-dominated health care regime, if physicians provided more services they made more money, and this played a large part in the run-up of health care costs in the 1980s.

Under capitation's fixed-payment system, however, more can be less for providers. Physicians were previously free of the burden of risk under the traditional indemnity insurance and fee-for-service arrangements, which paid them on the basis of costs, or charges (Weiner and de Lissovoy 1993). Under capitation, by agreeing to provide a set of medical services for a fixed annual or monthly payment per person, providers take on the financial risk of their decisions because capitated payments in essence represent a budget that physicians must manage (Berenson 1998). Providers thus have enormous incentives to control the volume of services provided to remain within the preset limits (Reinhardt 1995).

A 1994 survey of managed care plans revealed that more than half of responding network or independent practice association-model HMOs and more than one-third of staff—or group—model HMOs relied on capitation as their main payment method for primary care physicians (Gold et al. 1995). A 1997 survey by the Center for Studying Health System Change found that 54 percent of responding physicians reported their practices received capitation for at least some of their patients. Capitated contracts represented one-third of the average doctor's salary in 1997 (Stolberg 1998).

Capitation is even less prevalent in the hospital sector, where capitated contracts are responsible for less than one-tenth of all hospital revenues (Fubini and Bush 1998). It is unclear whether capitation will become increasingly more common, given concerns regarding its impact on quality, as well as uncertainty over how capitation will fare as greater numbers of higher risk patients are brought under managed care's umbrella (Berwick 1996).

One change that is occurring within some plans is the shift of capitation payment arrangements from primary care physicians to specialists. The rationale is that specialists provide the larger share of expensive health care services yet are still paid on a fee-for-service basis; by placing specialists under a capitated arrangement, it is hoped that more cost control leverage can be brought to bear on those responsible for the lion's share of expenditures. Plans may come to feature a mixture of discounted fee-for-service for primary care physicians and capitation for certain specialties—particularly those where there is an oversupply of physicians and where a large amount of relatively low-cost services are provided such as radiology, laboratory, and orthopaedics (Berenson 1998).

MANAGED CARE AS EFFECTIVE AGENT OF COST CONTROL

We have seen how the growth of managed care has transformed the health care landscape, changing how services are delivered, how providers are paid, and in many cases how they are forced to bear the financial risk for their decisions. The widespread shift into managed care has also brought about a dramatic reduction in the rate of growth of health care spending. As described previously, national expenditures on health care grew at a torrid pace throughout the 1980s and into the early part of the following decade. By 1993 the fever had broken, as the annual rate of growth averaged slightly more than 8 percent. But that was only the beginning: By 1996 the growth rate of health spending hit an all-time low of 4.4 percent—the smallest increase in four decades (Figure 2–8).

From 1989 to 1996 private-sector spending grew at an average annual rate of less than 6 percent, compared to twice that rate over the 1975 to 1989 period. Public sector spending did not enjoy as dramatic a decrease in growth rates, however, dropping from an 11.5 to a 9.7 percent average growth rate over the same time period. Such contrasts serve to explain the concerted efforts to extend managed care's reach deeper into the Medicare and Medicaid programs (Levit et al. 1998).

Managed care has certainly been the answer to employers' cost-control dreams, as it appears that they have finally broken the back of the health care cost inflation monster. Government figures indicate that the annual growth rate of private health insurance premiums plummeted from more than 18 percent in 1990 to less than 4 percent in 1996 (Figure 2–9).

The real annual rate of increase in health insurance premiums—which is to say the premium growth rate adjusted for inflation—has actually fallen below zero in recent years. And whereas there was significant difference in real premium growth rates among traditional indemnity, PPO, and HMO plans in the late 1980s, by the early 1990s real rates of growth had converged markedly (Figure 2–10).

Though managed care's impact on slowing cost increases is certainly impressive and should not be downplayed, two other contributing factors

FIGURE 2-8   National Health Expenditures, 1970–1996

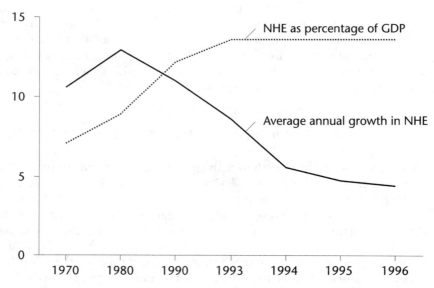

Source: Health Care Financing Administration, Office of the Actuary, National Health Statistics Group, quoted in Levit et al. 1998. "National Health Spending Trends in 1996." *Health Affairs* 17, no. 1.

must be considered. The first is the impact of the proposed Clinton health reforms: Though never enacted, the Clinton administration's proposals put fear in the hearts of the health care industry, which fought hard to stave off government regulation by controlling costs on their own. Indeed, this was a pattern witnessed throughout recent history: Reforms proposed by Presidents Nixon, Carter, and Reagan were accompanied by a marked slowdown in health care cost increases, only to be followed by a return to previous rates of growth (Thorpe 1997).

In addition, the slowdown in health spending increases was aided by a booming economy that virtually soared out of the 1991 recession with record growth rates and low rates of inflation. Strong economic growth enabled national health expenditures to remain steady as a share of GDP from 1993 to 1996.

COSTS: WHAT GOES DOWN MUST COME UP

It is not clear whether U.S. health care costs will remain in check. Indeed, there are several compelling reasons why they probably will not. First, many managed care companies have kept their prices artificially low to in-

FIGURE 2-9   Employer-Sponsored Private Health Insurance Premiums, 1990–1996
(percentage of change)

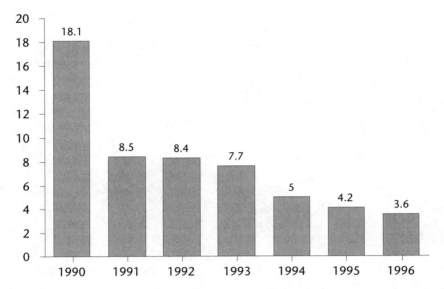

Source: Health Care Financing Administration, Office of the Actuary, National Health Statistics Group, and Office of Personnel Management, quoted in Levit et al. 1998. "National Health Spending Trends." *Health Affairs* 17, no. 1.

Note: Totals include employer and employee shares of premiums

crease their market share. As a result, more than 90 percent of for-profit managed care plans were profitable in 1994–1995, but less than 40 percent were in 1996–1997 (Ginzberg 1997a). These companies have Wall Street investors to answer to, and must now focus on generating profits. Moreover, it is widely recognized that to better manage care, plans need bigger and better information systems; weak profit margins curtail their ability to invest in such systems (Anders 1998).

Premiums for employment-based health insurance had increased more slowly than both medical and overall inflation over the past several years. In 1998, however, premiums rose 3.3 percent after rising only 2.1 percent in 1997, surpassing rates of both medical and overall inflation (Figure 2–11). Though these increases were below what many observers had predicted, observers expect premiums to continue to rise. The Congressional Budget Office estimates, for example, that premiums will rise at an annual rate of 5 to 6 percent over the next decade.

Second, experts note that managed care has already taken advantage of the "easy savings" by trimming payments to providers and by reaping the one-time savings engendered by the widespread shift of employees

FIGURE 2-10   Real Annual Growth in Premiums per Health Plan, 1987–1996
(percentages)

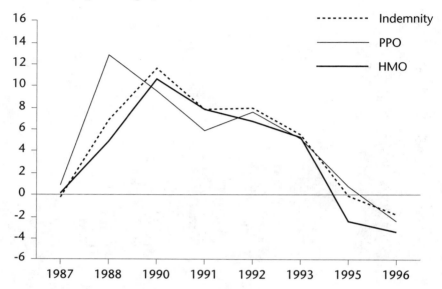

Sources: GAO calculations based on data from KPMG Peat Marwick (1991–1996); HIAA (1987–1990), and BLS consumer price index. Includes employer and employee shares of premiums for workers in private firms with at least 200 employees. U.S. GAO. 1997. *Employment-Based Health Insurance: Costs Increase and Family Coverage Decreases.* Washington, D.C.: U.S. Government Printing Office.

from fee-for-service into managed care plans. With more than 80 percent of the population in managed care already, fresh recruits are scarce. The one growth area for managed care plans is among higher risk, higher cost beneficiaries. Yet it is unclear whether Medicaid managed care, for example, will be capable of controlling costs while providing coverage for elderly and disabled individuals and chronically ill people, who represent nearly two-thirds of total Medicaid expenditures (Ginzberg 1997a).[17]

Third, other factors that will likely contribute to higher health care costs are the aging of the population, constant advances in—and public demand for—expensive medical technology, rapidly rising prescription drug costs,[18] physician consolidation, and patients' demands for regulation to ensure expanded access and higher quality health care services.

---

[17] Indeed, cost pressures are causing major HMOs to discontinue their Medicaid programs in several states (Langreth 1998).

[18] Prescription drug expenses for managed care plans increased 34 percent per member per month between 1993 and 1996 (Levit et al. 1998).

FIGURE 2-11   Health Insurance Premiums and Inflation, 1995–1998 (percentage increase)

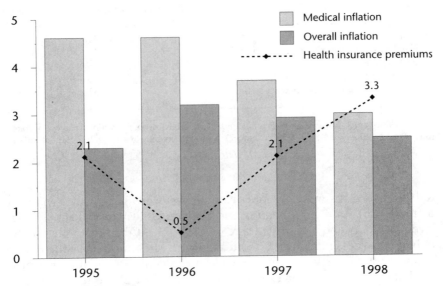

Source: KPMG Health Benefits in 1998.

Serious financial instability in the Medicare program overall, and expected cuts in Medicare's reimbursement rates for Medicare HMOs, combined with the continued cost shifting (albeit reduced) associated with the growing numbers of uninsured, will put upward pressure on health care costs (Fisher 1998; Hilzenrath 1998b). Continuing excess capacity despite managed care's efforts to squeeze the fat from the health care system—acute care hospitals are currently operating at 60 percent of capacity (and as low as 40 percent in some areas)—will serve as a counterweight to upward pressures, as will employers' ongoing dedication to holding down health care costs (Ginsburg and Gabel 1998; Ginzberg 1997a).

MANAGED CARE UNDER FIRE

At the same time that managed care's ability to control costs on a sustainable basis is being questioned, it also faces a considerable backlash from consumers and physicians alike. Patients' concerns center on whether the plans are more interested in cutting costs and making profits than delivering high-quality care, and on the perception that plan doctors' compensation is closely linked to how much they limit services and contain costs.

TABLE 2-2   Americans' Views on Managed Care

Managed care	Percentage of respondents agreeing
Decreases quality of care	51
Is more concerned with saving money than the best medical treatment	55
Makes it harder to see specialists	59
Reduces time doctors spend with patients	61

Source: The Henry J. Kaiser Family Foundation and Harvard University National Survey of Americans' Views on Managed Care, 1997 (November). Menlo Park, CA: Kaiser Family Foundation 1997 (November).

A 1997 national survey on Americans' views of managed care conducted by the Kaiser Family Foundation and Harvard University indicated a high level of anxiety about managed care (Table 2-2). At the same time that the public is expressing concern about managed care's impact on the quality of and access to services, there is widespread confusion about what managed care actually is. For example, more than half of the respondents to the Employee Benefit Research Institute's 1998 health confidence survey responded that they had never been in managed care—even though they were enrolled in a managed care plan at the time (Fronstin and Hicks 1998). This lack of understanding about managed care plans likely feeds consumer dissatisfaction with the plans. Finally, research indicates that individuals who are not given a choice of health plans are the most dissatisfied with managed care (Gawande et al. 1998). Currently, 44 percent of medium and large employers offer one health plan to their employees, and in smaller firms (200 employees or less) the share rises to 80 percent (Kaiser Family Foundation 1998).

Health care providers are also part and parcel of the managed care backlash, reacting to the constraints placed on their autonomy as well as their income by the constant pressure to trim costs. Providers have responded to these pressures in several ways. First, anecdotal evidence indicates that increasing numbers of the most senior, highly experienced physicians are leaving the practice of medicine at earlier ages. Whereas physicians might once have worked until they could physically no longer practice, many now are fleeing the medical profession as soon as they feel financially comfortable. Second, increasing numbers of physicians are applying for disability benefits, and declining morale is cited as a key factor in this trend. Third, physicians eager to reclaim control and clinical autonomy have attempted (unsuccessfully) to unionize to form countervailing power against the HMOs. Physicians and hospitals are forming their own delivery systems to compete head on with managed care companies.

The backlash against managed care has fueled a legislative jugger-naut; state legislatures introduced more than 1,000 managed care reform bills in 1996, and most states currently have one or more "consumer pro-tection" laws on the books, such as restrictions of so-called gag rules that were perceived to limit physician communication with patients and re-quirements for plans to cover emergency room treatment if a "prudent lay person" determines that such care is necessary.

On the national level, strong regulatory measures aimed at managed care were debated throughout 1997–1998 but none ever passed. Proposed national regulatory measures that were considered included requiring speedier access to specialists and disclosure of more information to con-sumers; allowing patients to sue their health plans (anathema to many Republicans who have sought to limit medical malpractice awards); and banning health plans from paying bonuses to doctors, hospitals, or claims adjusters for limiting patients' care (McGinley and Cummings 1998; Neal 1998).

Opponents claim that regulatory measures would result in increased premiums, rising numbers of uninsured, and would render employers vul-nerable to lawsuits. Yet public opinion polls indicate significant support for some form of legislated patient protection. The Henry J. Kaiser Family Foundation's national survey of Americans' views on managed care re-vealed that 52 percent of respondents in 1997 said government should protect managed care consumers; this increased to 65 percent in the 1998 poll. It is interesting to note that support for some form of regulation does not appear to be the result of Americans' initial reaction to a new health care marketplace featuring managed care; California has the longest run-ning relationship with managed care and the answers of respondents from California do not differ markedly from those of the United States as a whole. Public support for government intervention drops markedly, how-ever, when respondents are told that it would raise health care costs.

Three of the household names in the nonprofit health care arena—Kaiser Permanente, Health Insurance Plan of Greater New York, and Group Health of Puget Sound—have endorsed federal regulation of managed care (Kuttner 1998). The 1997–1998 debate over patients' rights broadly de-fined is likely to be revisited in the 107th Congress and may be a harbin-ger of increased governmental attention to perceived problems in the man-aged care arena (Carney and Serafini 1998; Goldstein and Neal 1998).

THE FUTURE: INCREMENTAL APPROACH
AS THE ONLY GAME IN TOWN

The short life of the Clinton health reform plan marked "the end of an era" in the long-running debate over extending access to the entire population

(Aaron 1996a). Indeed, Clinton's "big bang" reform (Klein, 1995) was *too* big for the U.S. public, businesses, and the vested interests of the trillion-dollar U.S. health care system. Its demise sent the pendulum swinging away from the massive overhaul side of the reform spectrum. The 1994 Republican takeover in Congress dealt the final blow to attempts to enact sweeping reform measures, and locked the United States even more firmly into the incremental camp of health care reform.

Piecemeal legislation that has been dubbed alternately "body-part legislation" and "disease-of-the-month legislation" has included such measures as requiring health plans to cover a minimum number of days in the hospital after a woman gives birth and extra days in the hospital for mastectomy surgery (Serafini 1997a). Mental health parity legislation enacted in 1996 forbids insurers from imposing dollar limits on mental health care services that are lower than those for physical health care services. The Health Insurance Portability and Accountability Act (HIPAA) was enacted in 1996 to address problems faced by individuals and those in the small-group insurance market in obtaining coverage, including issues such as guaranteed issue and renewal, limits on preexisting condition exclusion clauses, and portability. HIPAA requires insurers to make policies available to people who had lost their coverage after they lost their jobs.[19] The Children's Health Insurance Program (CHIP) enacted in 1997[20] was the largest expansion of health insurance for children since the enactment of Medicaid in 1965 (Ginsburg 1998). The program is designed to provide coverage to a large share of the uninsured population—namely the more than 10 million under age 18 who are not eligible for Medicaid.

Even with the establishment of these new programs, the problem of declining access looms large and will likely grow as health care costs begin to climb. Incremental programs will have some impact, but are akin to "shoveling sand against the tide," as pointed out by Drew Altman, president of the Henry J. Kaiser Family Foundation (reported in Pear 1998). Currently, more than 43 million Americans lack health insurance coverage, up from 38 million in 1992 when the problem of the uninsured was one of the primary targets of Clinton's health care reform effort (Figure 2–12). Estimates indicate that that number will approach 50 million by 2005 (Fronstin 1998b; Thorpe 1997).

Employment-based insurance covered 69 percent of the population under age 65 in 1987 and 64 percent today. Other changes that will likely deepen the pool of uninsured: Employer-sponsored coverage for employee dependents has been dropping steadily, and employers have been shifting

---

[19] HIPAA did not, however, mandate that insurers had to make those policies affordable. GAO (1998b) recently reported that insurers were charging excessive rates—as high as 140 percent to 600 percent of the standard premium—for individual policies.

[20] The State Children's Health Insurance Program is Title XXI of the Social Security Act.

FIGURE 2-12   A Growing Problem: Nonelderly Americans without Health Insurance, 1987–1997

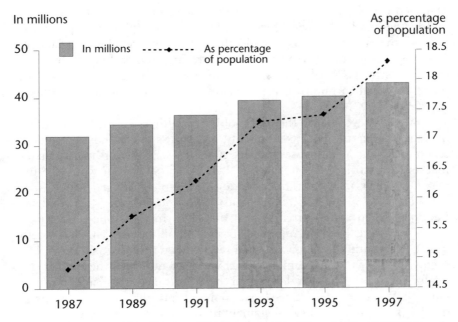

Source: Paul Fronstein, 1998. "Sources of Health Insurance and Characteristics of the Uninsured: Analysis of the March 1998 Current Population Survey." *EBRI Issue Brief. No. 204* (December).

a larger share of the burden to employees to the point where larger numbers of employees are turning down coverage because they cannot afford it (Cooper and Steinberg Schone 1997; U.S. GAO 1997a).

The problem of the growing numbers of uninsured must seem odd to people from many other countries: One might reasonably assume that because the relationship between insurance coverage and employment is particularly close in the United States, the uninsured would tend to be the unemployed. Given the booming U.S. economy and low rates of unemployment, one would reasonably expect coverage rates to increase, not decline. None of these assumptions translate into reality: More than one-half of the U.S. uninsured are working adults, generally low paid, either self-employed or working for a company with fewer than 25 employees.[21] Smaller companies are far less likely to provide health insurance to their employees than larger companies; approximately one-half of all companies with 50 or fewer employees provide insurance coverage to their workers.

---

[21] The typical uninsured person in the United States today is between the ages of 19 and 39, has children, an annual household income of between $40,000 and $60,000, and is a contingent worker in a small business in the service sector (Thorpe 1997).

IT AIN'T OVER YET

Managed care has, to its credit, put the brakes on health cost increases, and in the words of David Mechanic, brought "discipline to a pattern of practice that at the margins provided little value for the money"; removed the "incentives for overutilization of care and temper[ed] technological aggressiveness"; restored "the role of the primary care physician and offers potential to improve health maintenance and preventive services" (Mechanic 1997).

But all is not well in the house of U.S. health care. The fact that fundamental concerns about cost, quality, and access persist raises questions about what the next phase will be. After a decade's worth of dramatic market-led restructuring in the U.S. health care system, it would be unwise to believe that the transformation is complete; indeed it is best to consider the U.S. health care system as a "work in progress" (Ellwood and Lundberg 1996). We currently find ourselves in the "where do we go now?" phase; as health economist Marilyn Moon noted, "This is a wacky period in health care" (quoted in Freudenheim 1998d). Although it is highly unlikely that the United States will ever return to the unmanaged fee-for-service regime that dominated the U.S. health care system until the late 1980s, managed care itself faces significant challenges in terms of quality issues as well as the sustainability of its cost-control success.

Some observers predict the next phase of the managed care revolution may feature the replacement of the middlemen (the managed care companies) by employers contracting directly with providers for their services (Ginzberg 1997a; Hilzenrath 1998b; Iglehart 1996; Samuelson 1998). Direct contracting by employers was pioneered by the Buyers Health Care Action Group (BHCAG) of Minneapolis/St. Paul, an employer coalition of thirty-eight member employers in four states with more than 400,000 enrollees. In 1995 the BHCAG switched from joint purchasing of health care services from large health plans to direct contracting with doctors and hospitals aligned in what are known as "care systems."

It remains to be seen whether provider groups will be more successful than managed care plans at providing quality health care at reasonable cost. Regardless of whether it is provider groups or managed care plans that dominate the delivery system, the issue of quality is at the forefront; surveys indicate that people are more concerned about health quality than cost. Though the definition of *quality* as well as the appropriate ways to measure it is still open to debate, existing quality assessment tools include patient satisfaction surveys, report cards, and data sets such as the Health Plan Employer Data and Information Set (HEDIS), which contains performance measures that some employers use to evaluate health plan performance.

To paraphrase Mark Twain, news of health care reform's demise is greatly exaggerated. The ongoing problems masked by managed care's cost control success and a strong economy—such as concerns over the potential rise in health care costs for employers and consumers, growing anxiety over the quality of care, and increasing numbers of Americans without coverage—may provide the spark that will reignite the debate over national health care reform. The next phase of the debate will likely feature discussion of the appropriate role of the government in the health care system; the balance between regulation and health plans' and providers' autonomy; ways to expand coverage to the uninsured; how to ensure quality care and greater choice of health care plans and providers while controlling costs in an environment that features an aging population, and ongoing advances in medical technology. The debate should also revisit what the United States as a society expects from our health care system, what we are willing to pay, and whether access to health care coverage should be guaranteed to all as a right of American citizenship.

CHAPTER 3

German Health Care: Bismarck's Grand (and Enduring) Design

Germany established universal health insurance more than a century ago. Bismarck's grand design has served as a model for other nations, most notably the Netherlands and Japan. As one observer noted, the German system is the "original to which all other [health care systems] should be compared" (White 1995, 72).

Born in the shadows of the Industrial Revolution, the German health care system has shown remarkable resilience: It survived two world wars, the subsequent division of the nation into two distinct parts, and finally reunification in 1990. It has emerged from the traumas of history virtually intact and continues to be a popular fixture of contemporary Germany, which features a combination of a free-market economy and extensive social welfare programs (Kirkman-Liff 1990). The German health care system is a prominent component of this system of "capitalism with a heart" (Range and Livingston 1996).

German health insurance is characterized by its collectivization—all those earning below the government-specified income limit (currently approximately $43,000 per year[1]) are mandated by federal law to become members of a "sickness fund," which is a nonprofit health insurance organization. Only those whose incomes are above the ceiling are allowed to opt out of the system, and not everyone who has the option exercises it.

The sickness funds represent the patients in their dealings with health care providers, collect premiums in the form of employee and employer-paid contributions, and pay regional associations of providers from these revenues. Physicians are paid on a fee-for-service basis based on a negotiated regional fee schedule—not a nationwide fee schedule, as in Japan. The German system is known as an "all-payer system," because

---

[1] This amount refers to the limit in the western states; in the eastern states it is approximately $36,000.

all of the primary sickness funds in the same region pay providers the same fee for the same service.[2]

The importance of collectivization is evident in the legal requirement that all physicians and dentists practicing under the sickness fund system join an organization of sickness fund physicians. These sickness fund physician associations are different from professional trade associations such as the American Medical Association because of the sickness funds' legal authority to control the process of physician payment, as well as to monitor the services provided by physicians within their region (Schneider 1991).

The sickness funds themselves are also organized on a regional basis. Regional associations of sickness funds negotiate with the regional organizations of sickness fund physicians to set payment rates for ambulatory medical services. The key roles played by these two groups—the physicians' organizations and the associations of sickness funds—distinguish the German health care system from the health care systems of other nations (Hurst 1991; Schneider 1991).

OVERVIEW OF THE GERMAN HEALTH CARE SYSTEM

The German system's universal coverage[3] and comprehensive benefits combined with cost-containment success caught the eye of health policy experts during America's brief flirtation with national health care reform in the early 1990s. The proposed Clinton health care reform plan featured such elements of the German system as an employer mandate, payroll tax-based premiums, and large regional insurance groups.

The German health care system is situated toward the midpoint of the health system continuum. Health services are financed through income-related contributions paid by employers and employees, and the delivery system features a mix of public and private providers. The government essentially has a regulatory/oversight role rather than serving as a direct owner/provider of services. The government's presence is most evident in three major areas: (1) delineating broad legal parameters within which the system operates; (2) acting as the final arbiter in deadlocked negotiations; and (3) financing capital expenditures for the hospital sector (Reinhardt 1981b).

Consensus among the public and private sectors in the health care system is the glue that holds the system together (Anderson 1989). Basically, the government sets the overall framework and establishes the

---

[2] The substitute funds, which cover approximately one-third of all insured, negotiate their fees on a nationwide rather than regional basis. Physicians charge privately insured patients higher rates than sickness-fund insured patients.

[3] Fewer than 1 percent of the population is uninsured.

rules—in particular it ensures universal access by requiring employers to help finance health insurance coverage for their employees and by requiring employees earning below a certain income level to join a health insurance fund. The government also spells out what is contained in the comprehensive package of benefits covered by the national system and regulates the sickness funds, to the point that they can be more accurately described as quasi-public groups.

The German health care system accords much autonomy and responsibility to associations representing the physicians and the sickness funds, and the government historically has remained on the sidelines, allowing these groups wide latitude. Indeed, self-regulation *by* these groups and collective negotiations *between* them has been the norm, rather than governmental intervention. But determined cost-control efforts beginning in the late 1980s and continuing into the new century have resulted in a more interventionist role on the part of the government in the health sector and a consequent shift in power from the associations of payers and providers to the government (Schwartz and Busse 1997).

HEALTH CARE EXPENDITURES, THEN AND NOW

As of the mid-1970s and into the early 1980s, Germany and the United States dedicated nearly the same amount of resources, as a percentage of gross domestic product (GDP), to health care. But Germany implemented significant cost-control measures that effectively reined in health care expenditures to around 8 percent of GDP throughout the 1980s, while U.S. expenditures soared to 13 percent of GDP (Figure 3–1). Germany did such an effective job of containing costs that its health-to-GDP ratio actually declined from 8.4 percent in 1980 to 8.1 percent in 1990, the result of a national health care cost-containment policy that links growth in health care expenditures to increases in wages and salaries.

Germany's health care expenditure success came to a grinding halt shortly after the Berlin wall came crashing down; its famed cost-control magic lost the edge to the more powerful and now familiar litany of cost-inflating pressures of increased public demand for all the best the medical world had to offer, as well as a rapidly aging population. More than 16 percent of the German population will be age 65 or older by the year 2000, and more than 20 percent will reach this point by 2010 (Table 3–1).

If these factors were not enough, the tremendous ongoing costs of German unification—compared by one analyst to the United States absorbing all of Mexico (Sullivan 1993)—have exacerbated an economic slump featuring declining foreign investment and double-digit rates of unemployment. The former East German nation, formally dissolved on October 3, 1990, had a centralized, publicly owned and operated health care system.

FIGURE 3-1   Health Care Expenditures as a Percentage of GDP, U.S. and Germany, 1971–1997

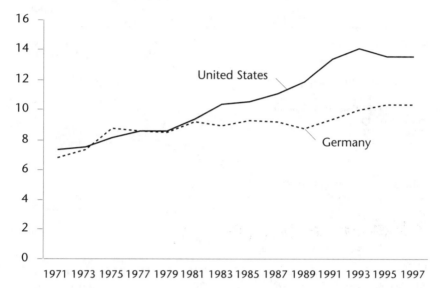

Source: OECD Health Data 98: A Comparative Analysis of 29 Countries. Paris: OECD/CREDES.

Most of the population was covered through the Free German Trade Union Federation, the primary organization for social insurance, and health care was lumped together with social security and funded through payroll and general tax revenues. Physicians were salaried state employees and hospitals were owned by the state (Hurst 1991; Stone 1991; Swabey 1990).

The merging of the very different social systems of the former "rich and poor cousins"—most of the more than 16 million residents of the former East Germany are poor relatives to their former West German neighbors—has required Germany to spend approximately $100 billion a year. Income levels are gradually increasing in the east and now approach 80 percent of income levels in the west; when they reach 90 percent the two health systems will be formally merged.

Combined employer–employee contributions for generous health, retirement, and unemployment benefits add more than 40 percent onto the cost of labor; at $31 an hour for manufacturing workers, Germany's labor costs are among the highest in the industrialized world and have made firms wary of setting up operations in Germany. High levels of unemployment[4] have a particularly deleterious effect on the financial position

---

[4] Unemployment in the former eastern states rose from 15 percent in 1992 to 21 percent in 1998; in the west from 5 percent in 1991 to 10 percent in 1998.

TABLE 3–1   Health Care in Germany and the United States

	United States	Germany
Life expectancy at birth	72.7 (male) 79.4 (female)	73.6 (male) 79.9 (female)
Median age of population	35	38
Projected percentage of population over age 65 in		
2000	12.5	16.2
2010	13.6	20.2
2020	17.5	22.5
Health care expenditures, 1997		
as percentage GDP	13.6	10.4
per capita	$4,090	$2,339
Distribution of health care spending, 1996–1997 (as percentage of total spending)		
Hospitals	34	35
Physicians	20	16
Drugs	9	13
Physicians per 1,000 persons, 1994	2.6	3.4
Inpatient hospital beds per 1,000 persons, 1996	4.1	9.6
Average length of stay (days), 1995	8.0	14.2
% of population admitted, 1995	12.4	20.7
Scanners per million persons, 1993	26.0	15.7
MRIs per million persons, 1995	15.5	4.8

Sources: OECD Health Data 98: A Comparative Analysis of 29 Countries. Paris: OECD/CREDES; World Bank.

of the health care system as it is financed through contributions in the form of payroll tax deductions.

Whereas health care expenditures as a percentage of GDP were held to a mere 1 percent increase over the 1982–1992 period, expenditures increased 28 percent from 1992 to 1996. Income-based premiums, which represented slightly more than 8 percent of salary in 1970, now average 13.5 percent (OECD 1998; Rublee 1998; Scholte and Doherty 1998).

The remaining sections of this chapter take a closer look at how the German health insurance system was developed and how it has evolved and expanded over its more than 100-year history. The first section examines the ideological and political underpinnings of the system that continue to shape German national health insurance, and later sections discuss health care financing and cost control in Germany.

PRESENT AT THE CREATION: TRACING THE ROOTS OF NATIONAL HEALTH INSURANCE

Social solidarity and the concept of a strong state were the guiding forces in the newly founded German Reich of the late nineteenth century (Blanpain, Delesie, and Nys 1978). Otto von Bismarck, chancellor of the imperial government—formed in 1871 through an alliance between the *Junker* (landed aristocracy) class and the Prussian military—devised the health insurance plan as a manifestation of his government's concern for the health of its citizens (Glaser 1983). The government was responding to new needs for social programs generated by the interrelated forces of "industrialization, population growth, urbanization, increasing wage dependence and the geographical concentration and political awareness of new industrial workers" (Zollner 1982, 5–9).

The importance of a strong state is firmly anchored in German history. As noted social historian Ralf Dahrendorf has pointed out, one of the peculiar features of German industrialization was a strong involvement on the part of the state in all aspects of the industrialization process—particularly in the area of workers' welfare (Dahrendorf 1976). That Bismarck would champion the first system of social insurance in Europe was quite consistent with his approach to government and industrialization and his view of the relationship between the state and society. Bismarck, according to historian Theodore Hamerow, "believed that government had a right to regulate the interaction of classes and interests for the advancement of the general welfare. He was never a doctrinaire supporter of individualism, whether in politics or economics." For Bismarck, "the preservation of the established order took precedence over the immunities and liberties of the citizen" (Hamerow 1973, 233).

Bismarck's response to the challenge of encouraging industrial development while at the same time preserving the political status quo was to bring about "reform from above"; the state would provide benefits as a means of ensuring workers' loyalty (Stone 1980, 21). Acting in his own political self-interest, Bismarck introduced "social rights to avoid granting wider political rights" (Starr 1982, 239).

Although Bismarck's advocacy of national health insurance in Germany stemmed from his belief in a strong yet benevolent state, it had overt political underpinnings as well. By offering health insurance to factory workers in the newly industrializing Germany, Bismarck hoped to make them loyal followers of the state and to preempt the growth of a nascent socialist party in Germany (Light 1985; Stone 1979). Bismarck believed that the only way to extinguish this movement was to fight fire with fire: Prove to the working class that the state would protect them so they would not be compelled to form trade unions or join the ranks of the Social Democratic Party (Blanpain et al. 1978). Not only would the new health insurance program give Bismarck healthy workers to staff Germany's factories, it would also ensure healthy soldiers for his armies.

1883 SICKNESS INSURANCE ACT

Business and labor groups fought against Bismarck's transparent attempt to consolidate his power. During the legislative debates following the introduction of proposals for health insurance in 1881, those groups strove to limit the reach of the federal government and to maintain "Germany's long tradition of autonomous groups" (Glaser 1983, 355). State legislators opposed federal attempts to take over responsibility for social programs, which they wanted to remain at the state level. Moreover, the existing mutual aid societies argued that they alone had the exclusive right to head the new insurance program (Light 1985).

These mutual aid societies were created by guild—and later union—members prior to the establishment of national health insurance. The societies, run by employers, employees, or both, collected dues from their members and in return provided access to medical services. Thus health care programs were run by societies on a local basis, funded by members' contributions. The concept of premiums was therefore not an alien one; workers were already paying premiums to these societies, and in some cases employers contributed some amount toward the total. The mutual aid societies facilitated the implementation of national health insurance, a new program built on an existing foundation (Light 1985).

The 1883 Sickness Insurance Act[5] required all workers earning a certain income or below (approximately 3 times the average wage at the time (White 1995)) be insured by a sickness fund or mutual aid society. The law also mandated employer–employee contributions (premiums) and stipulated a minimum level of benefits. The 1883 legislation guaranteed that all members of a sickness fund would receive physicians' services, medication, eyeglasses, and hospital treatment without charge at the point of service. Sickness funds were also required to provide income-replacement benefits, which were more important than medical benefits to workers at that time (Blanpain, Delesie, and Nys 1978).

---

[5] The Sickness Insurance Act was the first of three pillars of social security legislation in Germany, and was followed by accident insurance legislation in 1884 and old age and disability insurance in 1889.

Passage of the 1883 legislation was a success for Bismarck on two counts. First, social benefits for workers would be derived directly from an employment relationship, rather than from the state. The mode of financing health care through employer–employee contributions, rather than through general tax revenues was, and remains, a linchpin of the German health insurance system. Second, Bismarck's ability to draw health programs already in existence under the banner of the state as employer–employee organizations represented an effective check on the growing strength of the socialists and countered trade unions' efforts to be the exclusive source of social benefit protection (Lockhart 1981; Stone 1980).

Bismarck's social insurance system was based on the concept that a nation is responsible for the provision of social systems such as health care for its citizens. This "principle of social solidarity" essentially means that all members of society should have access to health care regardless of ability to pay, and that the costs of health care would be spread across the population. Hence, the reliance on income-based premiums (premiums based on what one earns rather than health risk) for health care financing means that wealthy individuals pay more than the less well-off (Iglehart 1991a; Wysong and Abel 1990).

GERMAN CORPORATISM

The final shape of the national health insurance program reflected both the social solidarity state-as-agent-of-social-welfare approach and earlier mutual-aid society arrangements. Although Bismarck did push through his version of national health insurance, he failed in his effort to secure a key role for the state governments in the administration of the program. That role fell to the sickness funds, which were similar to the mutual aid societies (Light 1985).

The "sickness funds compromise" was the embodiment of a particularly German organizational arrangement known as corporatism. German corporatism is characterized by a "quasi-public form of representative government over a specific program area" (Light 1985, 619) and stems from the belief that occupational groups are the best equipped to articulate political interests.

Two main features of German corporatism manifest themselves in the health care context. First, mandatory organizations whose membership is based on occupational status serve as intermediaries between the government and individuals. Second, these organizations are granted the legal authority to regulate "work-related aspects of their members' behavior and to administer government programs related to their members" (Stone 1980, 20). The compulsory organizations in this context are the sickness funds to which employees earning below a certain income must belong and the associations of sickness-fund physicians, of which any physician wishing to be paid under the sickness-fund system must be a member. The role of the state in this arrangement is to act as a referee with power to set the rules. The state can change the rules of the game through legislation if it feels that the system is off track (Light 1985).

The sickness funds were given legal responsibility over the financial and organizational aspects of health care services for their members. The funds were consequently responsible for staffing and operating medical facilities (Glaser 1978). The governing boards of the early sickness funds included representatives of employers and employees. Representation on the boards was in proportion to the share of premiums paid, and the unions volunteered to pay two-thirds of the premiums. The "resulting union control of the majority of seats would have a profound impact in the years to come" (Light 1985, 618), as the boards have always been responsible for determining such important factors as the size of premiums to be charged (Glaser 1983).

Unlike insurance premiums in the United States, risk factors are not a consideration in premium calculations. The German health insurance system thus had a redistributive bent from the start, as workers received similar (but not identical) benefits even though they did not necessarily contribute the same amounts (Glaser 1983). Through its income-based financing, the system enacts significant financial transfers between income groups, individuals with families and individuals without, healthy and sick alike (Wysong and Abel 1990).

SYSTEM EXPANDS

The 1883 law initially required manual laborers to join, but membership in the national health insurance system increased gradually over the years. Ten percent of the population was covered two years after the program's introduction. In 1911 the National Health Insurance Act increased the legal income limit for workers to be insured under the statutory program, and 23 percent of the population was insured by 1914. The number of insured has grown steadily since that time, to 28 percent in 1933, 48 percent in 1951, 85 percent in 1960, and approximately 90 percent of the population in 1998 (Henke 1990a; Schneider 1991; Statistisches Bundesamt 1998). Health policy expert Joseph White noted that this gradual expansion resulted in a "patchwork quilt" of insurance coverage rather than the "seamless garment of Canadian design" (White 1995, 73).

German national health insurance was implemented in the absence of opposition from doctors' groups (Anderson 1989). It was not surprising that physicians did not play a role in the initial formulation of national health insurance in Germany, because "they were not [then] recognized under law as a profession and did not have the extensive legal privileges of a profession" (Light 1985, 620). But as membership in the statutory system increased, private physicians came increasingly to believe their livelihood was being jeopardized by the stronger position of the sickness funds. Workers were attracted to clinics run by sickness funds because they were conveniently located and kept after-work hours. Each of the more than 20,000 different funds could specify which doctors would provide services to the funds members. Moreover, the sickness funds applied capitation (per person rates) or fee schedules to physician rates, which helped to contain costs (Light 1985; Zollner 1982). Thus the funds, by using closed panels to buy health care at a reduced cost, were acting in the capacity of early versions of modern American HMOs (Abel-Smith 1988).

The relatively weak position of physicians changed dramatically over the history of German national health insurance, as the doctors ultimately usurped the sickness funds to become the most powerful professional group in the health care sector (Light 1985). This trend began in 1900 with the founding of the Hartmann Bund, a physicians' organization dedicated to protesting the growing control of the sickness funds over the practice of medicine (Stone 1977). Indeed, as membership in the statutory health insurance program expanded after 1911, the number of funds decreased from 13,500 in 1914 to 6,600 in 1932. Physicians were thus confronted with larger organizations comprising larger patient constituencies (Stone 1980).

Thirty years after the formation of the Hartmann Bund, the Emergency Regulation of 1931 created associations of sickness fund physicians to represent those physicians participating in the national health insurance scheme. These physicians' associations were given the legal authority to negotiate fee schedules with the sickness funds as well as to conduct monitoring of physicians' practice. This granting of authority laid the groundwork for the evolution of physicians' organizations into very powerful political entities (Stone 1977). This also spelled the end of the early German HMOs because closed panels were effectively banned by government decree; no doctor was to have an exclusive contract or responsibility to any one fund. The funds could no longer serve as separate HMOs controlling the payment for health care services and making special deals with selected doctors because the regional associations of doctors was to negotiate physician payment terms. The elimination of these closed-panel organizations certainly casts a shadow over German efforts to implement features of U.S.-style managed care (Abel-Smith 1988).

THE CURRENT SYSTEM: HEALTH CARE BENEFITS, ORGANIZATION, AND FINANCING

The German statutory health insurance system has expanded over the course of its more than 100-year history, both in terms of population covered and scope of benefits. The system presents a unique approach to health care organization in its reliance on nongovernmental groups representing the insurers and the providers to administer the system, and financing remains dependent on premium contributions tied to income rather than risk status.

COVERED BENEFITS

The German health insurance program is among the most comprehensive in the world. Government regulations establish a basic benefits package that all funds must offer. Medical, dental, in-patient hospital care, prescription drugs, preventive care, and even rehabilitative treatments at health spas are covered. Patients do not pay deductibles, though there are minimal copayments for eyeglasses, dentures, prescription drugs, and the first fourteen days of a hospital stay.

Another measure of the breadth of German national health insurance is in the area of income replacement. Generous maternity benefits provide full pay during the period six weeks before birth through eight weeks after birth. The sickness fund pays a small portion of the allowance and the employer pays the bulk of the cost. If an insured person is unable to work because of an illness, employers are obligated to pay 100 percent of the employee's salary for up to the first six weeks of illness (Spencer and Associates 1999). According to health policy expert Christa Altenstetter, benefits such as these indicate that German national health insurance over the past century "has been fundamentally transformed into an all-inclusive health protection and income maintenance program for which the term 'insurance' may be a misnomer" (Altenstetter 1987, 507).

CORNERSTONE OF GERMAN HEALTH INSURANCE: THE SICKNESS FUNDS

The cornerstone of the German system is a network of approximately 700 health insurance funds known as *krankenkassen,* or sickness funds. Membership in the sickness funds is mandatory for all residents earning less than the government-established income ceiling of DM 6,375 per month (approximately $3,580)[6] in the former western states and DM 5,400 per month in the former eastern states. And, as in the U.S. Social Security program, only earned income up to this ceiling is taxable for health insurance. As the tax rate and the ceiling on taxable wages are fixed, an employee who earns $3,000 per month with four dependents, for instance, will pay the same amount as one without any dependents earning the same salary.

---

[6] Based on the exchange rate as of June 1, 1998, of 1.78 DM to $1 U.S.

In households in which both the husband and wife work, both contribute to their respective sickness funds. Approximately three quarters of the population earn below the income limit and are therefore mandated to be covered by the sickness fund insurance system, whereas an additional 13 percent of the population choose sickness fund insurance.

Up until the introduction of open enrollment in January 1997, an individual's employment determined which fund he or she joined, whether it was the fund set up by the employer, the fund covering the particular profession, or the local fund. Individuals who earn more than the income ceiling have the option of purchasing private insurance coverage, but only one in three chooses to do so. Private insurance rates are lower for those without dependents because the private insurers charge an additional premium for dependents, whereas the sickness funds do not. Restrictions prevent individuals from jumping back into the sickness fund system to take advantage of lower rates once they do have dependents; having opted out of the system, individuals are not allowed back in unless their income falls below the government-specified limit for mandatory coverage (White 1995; Wicks 1992).

The sickness funds have been likened to Blue Cross/Blue Shield groups in the United States, and are an example of what one expert calls "private socialism."[7] The funds are decentralized and governed by independent administrative boards, and are distinguished by their almost complete autonomy from both the federal (*Bund*) and the state (*Land*) governments. This mixture of federal mandate and decentralized administration is common throughout Europe (Henke 1990a).

Germany's sickness funds fall under two broad categories. So-called primary funds include local funds, which are the largest group of funds, providing coverage to 40 percent of the population (Figure 3–2). These local funds, known by the acronym AOK, tend to be the insurers of last resort, as they are obligated to cover individuals who do not belong to a particular employer group (OECD 1992). Primary funds also include company-based funds, which are set up by one employer for its employees and cover approximately 9 percent of the population; and trade and craft funds that cover specialized employee groups such as farmers, seamen, miners, and so forth.

The *Ersatzkassen* or substitute funds, whose predecessors were the early mutual aid societies discussed previously, cover nearly one-third of the population, and up until recently covered primarily white-collar workers.[8] As of January 1997, however, all Germans have free choice of insurance fund, as discussed in further detail later in the chapter.

---

[7] Uwe Reinhardt, cited in Sullivan 1993.

[8] The Germans have traditionally distinguished between white- and blue-collar workers.

FIGURE 3-2   Health Insurance Coverage, Germany 1995 (as a percentage of
              population)

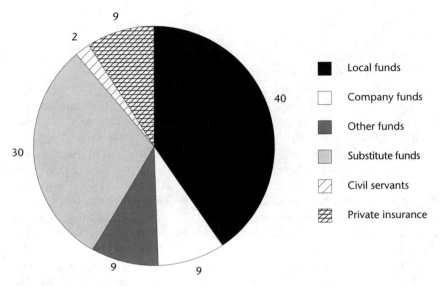

Source: Statistisches Bundesamt

Each sickness fund is supervised by a board of employee–employer representatives. Although these private nonprofit sickness funds are subject to federal guidelines, they are solely responsible for their own financial health (Reinhardt 1981b). The funds calculate the amount of revenues they will need to keep themselves solvent—including the cost of covering not only the insured members but their dependents, as well as all retirees covered by the fund—and set the employee–employer contribution rate accordingly (Iglehart 1991a).

In the early days of the sickness funds the ratio of contributions was two-thirds employees and one-third employer. This changed in 1951 when contributions were set at an equal level. An employee's contribution is not determined by risk status nor family status, because premiums are a set portion of income and cover all dependents (Reinhardt 1981b). It is interesting to note that though insurance premiums take the form of payroll taxes, they are not referred to as such, and are considered "contributions" to the universal health insurance system (Reinhardt 1993). And these contributions are not mere pittances; consider that an individual earning the equivalent of $36,000 would pay nearly $250 per month for health insurance coverage, with their employer paying an equivalent amount. This amount does cover all dependents and purchases a comprehensive package of benefits.

The sickness funds collect the contributions from their members and pay the regional physicians' associations, which then pay the doctors. In addition, with the advent of the new long-term care insurance program, the sickness funds are in charge of collecting and distributing the contributions for that program as well.

COVERAGE FOR THE SELF-EMPLOYED, RETIREES, THE UNEMPLOYED, AND OTHERS

Self-employed individuals generally purchase private health insurance, because they are only allowed to join a sickness fund if they had been a member of a fund before becoming self-employed. If they do join a sickness fund, they pay the entire contribution amount themselves.

Retirees receive benefits through their sickness funds—they remain members of the same fund they were members of at the time of retirement. A certain percentage of a retired person's public and private pensions—an amount equal to the average employee payroll contribution (currently nearly 7 percent of income)—is transferred to the sickness fund.

The unemployed and their dependents are protected by a federal law that requires sickness funds to provide the same benefits to the unemployed as to the employed. The Federal Labor Administration pays the premiums for the majority (two-thirds) of the unemployed, and the remainder of the unemployed are covered through local social welfare agencies (Iglehart 1991a). Although German health insurance is employment-based, loss of one's job does not necessarily entail loss of health insurance coverage—a significant problem in the United States.

Whereas the majority of civil servants are covered by the sickness fund system, 40 percent of civil servants are in a special category. These individuals, who tend to be high-level government employees and includes teachers are not allowed to join a sickness fund, and are reimbursed directly by their employer (federal, state, local government) for a portion of their health care costs, ranging from 50 to 95 percent. Most of the individuals in this group purchase private insurance to cover the cost of services not reimbursed by the government (White 1995; Wicks 1992).

As part of the agreement to restructure the former East German health system along West German lines, a network of sickness funds was created in the former eastern states in 1991.[9] Because of their low income levels, the vast majority of the population of former East Germany were required to join a sickness fund. Though contribution rates were set at the same average rate prevailing in the former western states, physician fees

---

[9] As of 1997 there were 56 sickness funds in the former eastern states. Only 2 percent of the population of the former eastern states had private insurance coverage as of 1995.

and hospital charges were to be set at a level of slightly less than half that in the west. These levels will gradually be increased as the gap between the standard of living in the east and west diminishes (Schneider 1991).

COMPANY-SPONSORED SICKNESS FUNDS

There has been a steady increase over the years in the number of health insurance plans sponsored by private companies. A little more than 400 employer-sponsored funds presently cover 9 percent of the population. Similar to self-insured plans in the United States, such company-sponsored plans are offered by larger employers and have a distinct cost advantage over the statutory sickness funds. Contributions tend to be lower because company-sponsored funds generally provide coverage for workers who are in lower-risk groups. In 1990, for example, the average contribution to company-sponsored funds was 11.1 percent of salary compared to 12.5 percent for the statutory funds.

The German government had grown increasingly apprehensive over the years about the number of company-sponsored plans, and was concerned that the funds increase the costs of the statutory sickness funds by attracting the lower risk enrollees. Indeed, one could argue that the availability of lower costs for only certain employers and employees belies the underlying principle of equality in German social policy. The German government's response came in the form of a risk equalization scheme in 1994, which is described later in the chapter.

OUTSIDE THE SICKNESS FUND SYSTEM: THE PRIVATELY INSURED

Germany has not outlawed private insurance for benefits covered under the national health insurance program; any individual earning more than approximately $42,000 per year can purchase insurance[10] from approximately forty-five private insurers. This alternative coverage represents to many the "escape valve for the affluent" that is absent in the Canadian system (U.S. GAO 1991). Slightly more than 13 million people had private insurance coverage in 1996, including 7 million individuals who were exclusively privately insured and 6 million who had supplemental private coverage (OECD 1997). The number of those exclusively covered by private insurance grew from nearly 5 million in 1980 to 6.6 million in 1990, and has since stabilized around the 7-million mark.

---

[10] Approximately 1 in 3 higher income earners choose private insurance.

Private insurance premiums are not income based but are adjusted for the age, gender, and health status of the insured at the time of enrollment. The premiums are designed to stay at a level amount, and do not increase as the individual ages or if he or she becomes sick. As a result, individuals pay more than actuarial cost when they are younger, thus setting aside a reserve needed to cover higher costs as they age (Iglehart 1991a; Reinhardt 1990a; Wicks 1992). Private insurance premiums are higher for married couples and families with children than sickness fund premiums because sickness funds do not charge extra premiums for dependents (Schneider 1991). If an employee opts to purchase private insurance rather than join a statutory sickness fund, the employer pays half the premium up to a maximum equal to the premium the employer would have paid if the employee had joined a statutory sickness fund (Reinhardt 1990; White 1995).

Privately insured individuals receive certain extra benefits, such as private hospital rooms and the right to be treated by the chief of a hospital department rather than the staff doctor. Providers charge private patients at rates that could be as high as twice that for sickness-fund insured patients. It is not widely believed that privately insured patients receive markedly better medical care (Knox and Straub 1993; Wicks 1992). Individuals purchasing private supplemental coverage generally do so to cover the cost of private or semiprivate hospital rooms, medical coverage during overseas travel, and coverage for dentures and eyeglasses.

LONG-TERM CARE INSURANCE PROGRAM

The sickness fund system provided some coverage for medical expenses for ambulatory care for the elderly, but in terms of long-term care expenses most of the elderly were forced to rely on their own private or family finances, or public welfare funds to cover the cost of such care. Indeed, the majority of individuals in nursing homes (0.5 million as of 1993) were on public assistance. Though private long-term care policies have been available since 1983, by 1993, for example, only 300,000 had been sold.

After nearly two decades of debate over how to finance long-term care, Germany introduced a public pay-as-you-go long-term care insurance program in 1995. The program is administered by the sickness funds; all those covered by the sickness fund system for health insurance are required to pay into the long-term care insurance program. Individuals covered by private health insurance are required to purchase a private long-term care insurance policy (Goerke 1996).

The program is financed through employer–employee contributions of 0.85 percent of pay. Employers long fought long-term care insurance, arguing that it was up to each individual to take out private insurance for such care. A compromise was reached when employees agreed to forfeit one paid holiday in exchange for employers' agreeing to pay half the contribution rate.[11]

Employers pay the same contribution amount for long-term care for those with private insurance coverage as they do for those with sickness fund coverage for long-term care. Everyone is covered under the long-term care system and everyone pays into it: The unemployed make contributions from their unemployment insurance and retirees pay through deductions of 0.85 percent of their private pensions and 0.85 percent of their social security pension checks (Spencer and Associates 1998).

The long-term care program covers home care as well as nursing home or other institutional care. The program was designed to provide a relatively limited amount of benefits, and the ceiling on expenditures leaves considerable room for private supplemental long-term care insurance policies to provide more comprehensive coverage.[12]

Private insurance companies are allowed to base their premiums on no other risk factors other than age, and their premiums cannot exceed the maximum premium charged by the sickness fund system (Goerke 1996). As of the end of 1996, Germany's two largest private health insurers had a combined 1.5 million long-term care insurance policy holders. The sale of supplemental policies—generally used to provide cash benefits—has increased 50 percent since 1995. Germany's largest private insurer currently provides 18,000 people with supplemental policies (Life Insurance International 1998).

HEALTH CARE DELIVERY

Health care services in Germany are delivered through a mixed public–private system. The majority of hospital beds are in pubic community hospitals run by state or local governments or universities, and physicians are either in private practice or are salaried employees of hospitals. Recent reforms have aimed to break down the seemingly impenetrable wall that divides office-based physicians' services from hospital-based services, with the goal of allowing hospital physicians, for example, to follow their pa-

---

[11] This does not apply to employees in the states of Sachsen and Schleswig-Holstein.

[12] The benefits amount vary according to need and severity of illness and are divided into three categories: medical goods and services are limited to DM 750, DM 1,800, or DM 2,800 per month, though in cases of extreme hardship payments can go as high as DM 3,750; cash benefits are limited to DM 400, 800, or 1,300 per month, depending on the illness, and payments for inpatient nursing are limited to DM 2,800 per month, or DM 3,300 per month for extreme hardship cases (Watson Wyatt 1998).

tients' progress after they are discharged from the hospital. The ultimate goal is to reduce lengthy hospital stays and eliminate costly duplication of services.

HOSPITALS

Hospitals in Germany are for the most part public institutions run by state and local governments, universities, or charitable institutions: 51 percent of all hospital beds are in public hospitals; 35 percent in private voluntary, often religious, hospitals; and the remaining 14 percent of all hospital beds are in private hospitals (Knox and Straub 1993). Germany has 9.6 inpatient beds per 1,000 population, high by U.S. standards (4.1 per 1,000), but down from the 1991 level of 10.1 beds per 1,000 (OECD 1998). Hospital-based physicians represent more than half of all physicians. Physicians in public hospitals are salaried employees of the hospital; doctors in private hospitals are paid on a fee-for-service basis.

Up until the early 1990s, hospitals were paid exclusively on a per diem basis, at a rate negotiated with the regional associations of sickness funds. Though physicians belong to associations of sickness fund physicians through which they negotiate fees, the 3,000 German hospitals negotiate the hospital budget, and from that the per diem rate, directly with the sickness funds.

All health care payers (sickness funds) in the same region pay the same per diem rate, regardless of the patient's illness (Henke 1986; Iglehart 1991a; Schneider 1991; Stone 1980). This payment system encouraged hospitals to keep their beds filled and led to excessively long hospital stays—14.2 days in 1995 (compared with 8 in the United States).

Hospital operating expenses are kept separate from capital investment funds. The latter were covered by federal and state government budgets, and operating expenses were included in the hospital per diem rate. The Hospital Financing Reform Law of 1984 put an end to this shared responsibility, however, and granted state governments the final say over the financing of all capital expenditures for medical facilities and equipment, effectively giving the states control over hospital capacity (Altenstetter 1987; Godt 1987; Jonsson 1990). Even private hospitals receive their capital investment funds from the state governments; this public financing spreads the financing over a wider base than the sickness funds alone, and reinforces the perception of hospitals as public utilities rather than private businesses (Knox and Straub 1993).

The 1984 law was followed by the Federal Hospital Payment Regulation of 1985, which instituted a prospective global budgeting system for hospitals. From that point forward, operating budgets were to be calculated in advance based on expected rates of hospital occupancy for the following year. Each hospital negotiates its budget with the sickness funds, and this results in a negotiated per diem rate paid by the sickness funds to the hospital (Altenstetter 1987; Hurst 1991; Schneider 1991).

Thus a dual system of hospital financing was created, with the state responsible for planning and investment in hospital capacity and the sickness funds responsible for hospital operating costs. Though this arrangement allows states to control expenditures on high-tech medical equipment, it makes for an uneasy alliance; states may not be sensitive enough to the impact of their decisions regarding capital expenditures, because they do not have to take responsibility for operating expenses. For example, although the states might purchase new equipment, they might not take into consideration the cost of operating the equipment that the hospitals will incur (Iglehart 1991b; Schneider 1991). The hospital payment system was significantly altered by the 1992 reform legislation, as discussed later.

PHYSICIANS

Excess capacity in the hospital sector has its corollary in physician supply: With 3.4 physicians per 1,000 population in 1995, Germany has one of the highest physician-to-population ratios in the world. The number of physicians nearly doubled between 1970 and 1990, even though the population remained at a steady level (Knox 1993). Measures have recently been introduced to control physician supply. Though unable to limit medical school placements because the constitution guarantees all citizens the right to free medical education, Germany has set up limits on the availability of physicians by region.

Most physicians are in private practice; though approximately one in five physicians are in group practices, the number has been growing (OECD 1997; White 1995). Twenty years ago general practitioners (GPs) dominated the physician landscape, but their numbers have declined to where they now make up approximately 40 percent of the physician population. Patients have free choice of physician, and the gatekeeper role of the GP is not well-developed; an estimated four out of ten patients do not go to a GP before seeing a specialist (Mullan 1998). Physicians in private practice still make house calls, typically to elderly patients.[13]

In Germany, as in many other European countries, there is a distinct legal separation of the services of ambulatory (office-based) physicians and hospital physicians. A physician is generally allowed to provide either

---

[13] A typical day for a primary care physician in private practice would consist of house calls between 7:30 and 9:00 A.M., office hours until 4:30, and then more house calls until 8:00 P.M. I am grateful to my colleague Mary Ellen Mullholand for pointing this out to me.

in-patient hospital care or office-based care only.[14] Though changes have recently been introduced to break down these barriers, in effect an office-based physician cannot treat his or her patient once that patient enters the hospital. In the same way hospital physicians are not allowed to conduct such prehospital procedures as diagnostic workups, nor are they allowed to provide follow-up care (Stone 1980).

All sickness fund physicians are organized into regional associations that negotiate fees with the sickness funds and pay the doctors. Each physician sends vouchers covering the type of service a patient received to the regional association of physicians for payment. These regional associations serve not only to pay physicians but also to monitor the volume of services performed by each physician. In this way the associations play a critical cost-containment role, as will be discussed more in following sections (Schneider 1991).

Physicians must accept payment from the sickness funds as payment in full. Again, as Germany has an all-payer system, all regional sickness funds pay the same fees for the same services to regional associations of sickness fund physicians. It should be noted, however, that private insurance pays physicians and hospitals at fee levels that are more than twice that of the sickness fund fee levels (Schneider 1991). And as noted earlier, the nationwide substitute funds negotiate fees on a national, rather than regional, basis.

EVOLUTION OF PHYSICIAN PAYMENT METHODS. Physician payment in Germany has evolved over the past several decades. The seeds of the current relationship between health care providers and payers were planted in 1931 and 1932, when physicians' associations were created to represent physicians in negotiations with sickness funds. Negotiations with individual physicians were no longer allowed and sickness funds were required to negotiate with physicians as a group (Kirkman-Liff 1990).

The 1931 and 1932 regulations also established a two-step physician reimbursement process. First, the sickness funds would make lump-sum capitation (per person) payments to the physicians' associations. The physicians' associations were then responsible for dividing this revenue pool and distributing individual payments to their physician members. These payments were generally made on a fee-for-service basis according to a fee schedule. The size of the pool and the specific fees for medical procedures were hammered out through collective bargaining between the physicians' associations and the sickness fund associations (Stone 1980).

---

[14] Chiefs of hospital departments alone are allowed to have private practices in the hospital to care for privately insured patients. The 1992 reform law contained provisions requiring hospital chiefs to pay a significant share—typically one-third—of what they earn from private patients to the hospital (Knox and Straub 1993).

Each physician's share of the total pool was determined by a relative value scale that applied a certain number of points to each medical service rendered. The total number of points accruing to each physician determined his or her share of the pool. The financial risk was thus spread among physicians because a sickness fund with a majority of low-income members would pay a lower capitation rate into the pool than a fund with mainly high-income earners. In this way the funds with wealthy members subsidized the funds with poorer members (Kirkman-Liff 1990).

The sickness funds contributed to the pools on a capitation basis for the next two decades, during which time a system of fixed budgeting essentially governed physician payment methods. But a 1955 reform empowered sickness funds to select their preferred method of calculating the pool: fee-for-service, fee-per-visit, capitation, or any mix of these (Stone 1980).

FROM CAPITATION TO FEE FOR SERVICE. The first sickness fund changed to a fee-for-service method of calculating the pool in 1958. The physicians' associations then staged a campaign that pitted the statutory sickness funds (which were still using the capitation method) against the substitute funds, which had made the switch to a fee-for-service method. The physicians' associations argued that as the statutory funds were still using a capitation method, the care they provided was of lower quality than the other funds. The statutory funds were therefore faced with loss of membership if they did not change to a fee-for-service method (Stone 1980). By 1968 the physicians' associations had succeeded in changing the payment system to a fee-for-service reimbursement system (Kirkman-Liff 1990).

Payments were made each quarter by the sickness funds to the regional physicians' associations; these payments were calculated by examining the claims in the previous quarter (Kirkman-Liff 1990). The limit on total expenditures for physicians' services was effectively wiped out by the new fee-for-service method of pool calculation. This new method allowed physicians to increase their share of the pie without detracting from that of their colleagues (Stone 1980). Indeed, the change from capitation to fee-for-service represented a significant windfall for physicians and would sound the death knell for efforts to control physician reimbursement.

TWENTY YEARS OF HEALTH CARE COST CONTROL: 1977–PRESENT

German health care expenditures rose from 6 to 8 percent of GDP from 1970 to 1975. The federal government turned to regulatory measures to combat such rapidly rising expenditures, and Germany became "one of the first countries to impose budgetary discipline upon national health insurance" (Glaser 1978, 111). Physicians in Germany were as enamored of government intervention as their American counterparts, yet despite their opposition, several landmark health care cost-control measures were enacted (Kirkman-Liff 1990).

HEALTH CARE COST CONTAINMENT ACT OF 1977

Germany took its cost-control mission seriously and formalized procedures—codified in the federal Health Care Cost Containment Act (HCCCA) of 1977—to rein in health care expenditures. This law was designed to reduce health care expenditure growth and create a framework for stabilizing the payroll tax rate for health insurance (Henke 1986). The law sought to introduce predetermined budgets for all health care expenditures (Reinhardt 1981a), and to that end created a national health conference (*Konzertierte Aktion*). The so-called Concerted Action is an advisory body made up of approximately seventy representatives of all the major shareholders in the health care system, including physicians, hospitals, dentists, as well as representatives of the pharmaceutical sector, employers, and labor unions.

The conference meets twice a year. Its mandate is to bring all the various groups together in an effort to work toward agreement on a uniform, nationwide, operational framework for the German health insurance system (Henke 1990a). All aspects of the system are discussed and negotiated, from overall expenditure levels to specific increases in physicians' fees. A key objective of the conference is the establishment of guidelines for the maximum annual increase in expenditures for physician and dental services and prescription drugs. Though the conference's guidelines are nonbinding, they do bear significant influence; if the groups are incapable of agreement, compulsory arbitration may be imposed (Kirkman-Liff 1990; Stone 1980). As health policy expert Joseph White explained, "The Concerted Action has no formal authority to set prices, rather it establishes a standard of reasonableness to which both negotiators and an arbiter might refer" (White 1995, 78).

A significant outcome of the 1977 legislation was a series of reforms that resulted in a new contract between the sickness funds and the physicians' associations. This contract established a target for physician expenditures. The target was calculated based on health costs for the previous year and could be adjusted to accommodate changes in demographics, new medical technology, and so forth. More important, the target was to reflect changes in wages and salaries of employees. This was the centerpiece of a new strategy known as income-related expenditure growth. Increases in expenditures would be tied to increases in the wage base of the sickness funds' members (Kirkman-Liff 1990; Schneider 1991).

In addition to establishing a target for physician expenditures, the 1977 law also formally established a national relative value scale (Godt

1987). Negotiations between the sickness funds and the physicians' associations were held on a national level to determine the point value assigned to more than 2,000 different medical treatments (Kirkman-Liff 1990). Whereas the relative value scale was negotiated between national associations of sickness funds and national associations of sickness fund physicians, the conversion factor used to arrive at a monetary equivalent for each point on the scale is set in annual negotiations between the regional associations of sickness funds and their physician counterparts. As a result, there is a series of regional fee schedules for physicians, but no single nationwide fee schedule (U.S. GAO 1991).

Conspicuously absent from the HCCCA were regulations affecting cost containment in the hospital sector. The hospital sector was able to elude the government's net as the states, which had primary responsibility for the hospital sector, wielded their veto power in the national parliament. It was not until 1982 that the hospital sector was formally included within the Concerted Action forum (Godt 1987).

The HCCCA was a watershed in the development of health care policy making in Germany, because it was the first time in many decades that the federal government directly intervened in the health care sector (Henke 1986). Whereas other reform attempts had failed, such as those undertaken in the 1960s to introduce cost-sharing, the successful implementation of the 1977 legislation can be attributed to three major factors. First, the public was well aware of escalating health care expenditures. Second, these health care costs were widely perceived to be jeopardizing the financial standing of the social security system. Third, public opinion was enraged by the wide disparity in income levels between physicians and other workers (Godt 1987; Stone 1980). Indeed, physicians' incomes were almost five to six times the national average wage from 1970 to 1975. The federal government, with strong public support for reform, was able to "mobilize a coalition of labor and business leaders [the primary financiers of the health care insurance system], who were hostile to the doctors' positions" (Godt 1987, 475).

1986: FROM EXPENDITURE TARGET TO CAP

Although the expenditure target appeared to be a plausible approach in theory, in reality health care expenditures during the period that the target was in use (1978–1986) always surpassed the target figure. Targets were essentially nonbinding; when spending exceeded the target, future expenditures were not reduced accordingly. Tighter control over physician expenditures was needed, and it was decided that an expenditure cap would be a more effective method of cost control. Expenditure caps were given the teeth that expenditure targets lacked and set binding limits on annual expenditures for physician services. Increases in the expenditure cap were directly linked to increases in the average wage level of sickness funds' members (Kirkman-Liff 1990).

The expenditure cap was set every year through negotiations between the sickness funds and the physicians' associations; a separate cap was set for three categories: basic services, laboratory services, and other services. Approximately one-fifth of all outpatient services was excluded from the cap; as these services were generally preventive in nature, it was decided that it was not appropriate that they be subject to the expenditure cap.

A certain amount of money was allocated for each person (capitation amount) insured by the sickness fund system; a total budget amount was determined by multiplying this figure by the number of insured. The sickness funds pay the physicians' association a lump-sum payment; the association then pays the doctors on a fee-for-service basis. Under the expenditure cap, when the volume of services exceeded the limit set by the cap, the point value used to determine physicians' fees was reduced.

As Reinhardt noted, the system of downward adjustment of fees made all physicians part of a "zero-sum-game" as they all drew from the same revenue pool. The physician associations consequently "police[d] their own members" (Reinhardt 1990, 9), monitoring physicians claims and treatment records to check for overservicing. Expenditure caps were designed to correct the weaknesses of the previous cost-control mechanism, because not only could the caps enforce spending limits but they contained a built-in mechanism to prevent physicians from increasing the volume of services to increase their incomes, given the bottom line that volume increases would reduce the value of the point used to determine the physicians' reimbursement rate. Though physicians were paid on a fee-for-service basis, they were never sure what the specific fee for each service would be, because it all depended on whether expenditures exceeded or remained under the cap (Knox 1993; Stevens 1992).

Yet even though the physicians were bearing the risk for expenditures that exceeded the cap, expenditures did continue to increase, a result in large part of the increasing supply of physicians. The caps did a better job of containing expenditures than the previous regime of expenditure targets. However, physician spending for outpatient services increased at a rate of 7 percent a year between 1977 and 1985; under the caps the increase was held to 2 percent a year (U.S. GAO 1991). But other sectors were not subject to the cap, and health care costs continued to rise faster than wages.

1989 HEALTH REFORM LAW

Concerns over rising health care costs continued into the late 1980s as employer–employee insurance contributions reached a high of nearly 13

FIGURE 3-3   Average Contribution Rates for Sickness Funds, 1970–1990 (as percentage of covered income)

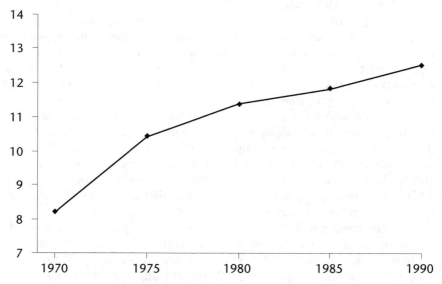

Source: Bundesministerium für Gesundheit, 1998

percent in 1988 (Figure 3–3), heightening anxiety that increasing contribution rates were inflating labor costs (already among the highest in Europe); it was feared that such high costs would ultimately render German industry uncompetitive. Moreover, the federal government was concerned that the continued increases in spending on health care might reduce any gains derived from a gradual reduction in income taxes (Goebel 1989).

The government passed the comprehensive Health Reform Law of 1989, which implemented a series of cost-control measures, including: doubling the copayment rate for each of the first fourteen days in the hospital from DM 5 to DM 10; instituting a copayment of DM 3 per prescription; increasing copayments for dental services; setting limits on reimbursement of transport and travel costs; eliminating funeral (death) grants for newly insured (such grants for those already insured were reduced); and eliminating lump-sum birth grants (Goebel 1989; Will 1989).

Among the more important aspects of the Health Care Reform Act was the creation of a reference price system for pharmaceuticals. This system grouped drugs into classes of therapeutic equivalence and set a reference price for each group of drugs. The reference price is set below the highest price drug in the group—usually the leading brand name drug—and above the lowest price drug—usually the generic. The sickness funds will not reimburse above the reference price; if a patient chooses a more expensive drug, they must pay the difference out-of-pocket. Initially, approximately half of all pharmaceuticals were covered under the reference price system, with the eventual goal of 70 percent of all drugs (GAO 1994). The prices of drugs with fixed rates were reduced by more than 20 percent in the first year of implementation of price controls (Schneider 1991).

These reforms were designed with the objective of shaving about 10 percent off the total German health care bill. The specific measures targeting the pharmaceutical industry, for example, were deemed critical. The Germans, like the Japanese, are heavy consumers of prescription drugs,[15] and drug prices in Germany were twice as high as those in any other industrialized country. Pharmaceuticals accounted for more than one-fifth of all health care expenditures at that time (Schieber, Poullier, and Greenwald 1991).

HEALTH CARE REFORM AS A PERMANENT STATE?

Even after implementation of the 1989 reform program, contribution rates continued their uphill climb, rising from 12.2 percent in 1991 to 13.4 percent in 1992. The government decided that it was time to stem the rising rates and introduced health reform legislation in the fall of 1992 that took effect in January 1993, a pace at which Americans could only dream of seeing legislation enacted (Knox and Straub 1993).

The Structural Health Care Reform Act of 1993 featured a series of bold cost control measures, which targeted not only physicians but other sectors as well: The doctors had carried the cost-control burden for years, whereas other sectors were virtually free to spend. The 1993 act changed all that. Its ambitious scope might qualify as an example of what Rudolf Klein has termed "Big Bang" health care reform (Klein 1995) and led to dire warnings of the end of Germany's vaunted consensus-driven national health care system and the beginning of "socialized medicine" under what was perceived to be the heavy hand of government.

The most significant feature of the act was the imposition of separate budget caps on each of the major health care sectors: outpatient physicians, hospitals, pharmaceuticals, and dental services. Though physicians and hospitals were already accustomed to budgets and expenditure limits, the dental and pharmaceutical sectors were to feel the weight of the cost-control hammer for the first time. The caps were designed to limit health spending to increases in workers' income—essentially tying expenditure

---

[15] See Lynn Payer (1996), *Medicine & Culture*, for an interesting discussion of the role of prescription drugs in the German health care system.

growth to the wages on which taxes are levied to finance the health care system—with the main goal of stabilizing the contribution rate.

In addition to capping all health care sectors to a 4 percent expenditure growth rate, the law increased copayments on pharmaceuticals and hospital stays; changed the way hospitals were paid; set limits on physician supply; set up a financial risk equalization scheme designed to narrow the difference in contribution rates among the sickness funds; and allowed individuals to choose, for the first time, which particular sickness fund they wanted to join. Each of these reform measures is discussed in turn.

A CAP FOR ALL SECTORS

The 1993 law put caps on health expenditures in the physician, hospital, dental[16] and pharmaceutical sectors, which were to be in place for the 3-year period 1993 to 1995, but actually remained in effect for several years longer. These caps limited the rate of expenditures to the income growth of the sickness funds members. The 1993 expenditure limit was set based on 1991 expenditure levels, plus growth in income in 1993; the 1994 limit was 1993 expenditures plus growth in income for 1994, and so on.

The pharmaceutical sector was a particularly visible target for expenditure control, because drug prices had risen 10 percent every year throughout the 1980s, and pharmaceuticals consumed one-fifth of all health care spending. The law put the onus of pharmaceutical cost control squarely on the physicians' shoulders by placing the physicians at financial risk for exceeding the cap. The 1991 pharmaceutical expenditures of DM 24 billion[17] was set as the 1993 spending limit. Any amount beyond the cap (up to a limit of DM 280 million) would reduce the following year's budget for physicians' services, and any excess beyond DM 280 million would come out of the drug makers' pockets through a reduction in drug prices. In addition, prescription levels of individual physicians would be monitored, and if overprescription occurred (prescribing more than 25 percent of the average) physicians would take a hit on their income through a deduction for any overruns (GAO 1994b; Henke, Murray, and Ade 1994).

In an effort to make consumers more aware of pharmaceutical costs, copayments were increased from a flat DM 3 to DM 3, 5, or 7 depending on the size of the prescription. The Reference Price System (RPS) established by the 1989 Health Care Reform Act had successfully encouraged physicians to prescribe less costly generic drugs. The 1993 reforms added

---

[16] In addition to a cap on expenditure growth for dental services, the law actually reduced reimbursement rates by 10 percent for dentures and orthodontic services and required dentists to give a two-year warranty on every filling.

[17] The caps were set at roughly $15 billion in 1993 dollars, a 9 percent cut from 1992 expenditure levels.

more cost-control muscle by requiring manufacturers to reduce the prices of drugs not in the RPS by 5 percent and the price of over-the-counter pharmaceuticals by 2 percent.

By the end of the first year of the caps, spending per sickness fund member fell more than 1 percent from 1992 levels (which had increased 10 percent from 1991 levels). All major sectors of the health care system experienced decreases in the rates of spending, particularly in certain categories such as pharmaceuticals, where spending per sickness fund member fell by nearly 20 percent, and dentures where spending per member fell by nearly 27 percent. As a result, contribution rates declined from 13.4 percent in early 1993 to 13.25 percent in April 1994 (GAO 1994a).

CHANGE IN HOSPITAL PAYMENT SYSTEM

The reform law also targeted the hospital payment system, whose per diem payment rate was, as noted previously, linked to excessively long hospital stays. The new system introduced patient management categories (PMC) defined around specific illnesses, somewhat akin to Medicare's diagnosis-related group (DRG) system. This prospective payment system would cover all hospital care costs for approximately seventy specific cases or diagnoses. Approximately 150 hospital interventions were costed out under separate procedure fees. More than one procedure fee could be charged per case. Other costs such as administrative overhead and room and board are covered under a hospital-specific basic daily rate. The new payment system was devised with the aim of eliminating the incentive to keep patients hospitalized for long periods of time, paying the hospital per procedure or case rather than according to how long a patient is in the hospital.

The law also contained measures to break down the walls between ambulatory and hospital care to reduce duplication of services by allowing hospital physicians to perform outpatient surgery and to care for patients for short periods before and after admission to the hospital.[18] The act allows hospitals to open ambulatory surgery departments, with the aim of reducing inpatient care and improving cooperation between the ambulatory and hospital sectors (GAO 1994a).

LIMITS ON PHYSICIAN SUPPLY

Germany is overdoctored, with 3.4 doctors per 1,000 population compared to 2.6 in the United States and 2.2 in Canada. Though the German government cannot cut back on the number of medical students—because all

---

[18] Hospital doctors will be able to provide three treatment days within five days of admission and seven treatment days within fourteen days of discharge.

qualified medical students have a constitutional right to state-subsidized medical education—the new law sought to reduce the number of practicing physicians through limits on licensing if there is more than 110 percent of the government-set limit on physician capacity in a certain region. As of late 1993, for example, physicians could not open new practices in large cities such as Hamburg and Munich (GAO 1994c). Such regional limits on physician supply have led to unemployment among physicians for the first time in Germany.[19]

The associations of sickness funds and sickness fund physicians have been charged with developing and implementing an allocation system for physicians and specialists based on population needs and availability of care. Moreover, as of 1999 a system of forced retirement will be introduced as all physicians age 68 and older will have their licenses revoked (GAO 1994a).

Prepare to Compete: The Financial Risk Equalization Fund

The 1993 reform law also introduced a method to narrow the range of contribution rates across the sickness funds in preparation for open competition among the sickness funds. Essentially, the risk equalization effort was a necessary precursor to competition based on quality of service and not risk selection.

In 1993 the average contribution rate was 13.4, with rates ranging from 8.5 to nearly 17 percent for a similar package of benefits. Given that sickness fund contribution rates are set according to the costs of covering all members of a fund, the varying composition of each fund—in terms not only of enrollees' ages, number of dependents, health status, but also of income levels—affects the rates the fund needs to charge. Funds that cover primarily lower income, higher risk workers must charge higher contribution rates to generate sufficient revenues to cover the costs of health care for their members (Rublee 1992). The local funds, which tend to be the insurers of last resort, have higher payroll tax rates. In 1993, for instance, the average tax rate of the local funds was 14.05 percent, whereas the average substitute fund tax rate was only 13.18 percent (Figure 3–4).

To determine whether a fund will pay into the risk pool or receive subsidies from it, two sets of calculations are performed. First the financial position of the particular sickness fund is determined by figuring out the total amount of income the fund has at its disposal (in other words, its payroll tax revenues) and then dividing this total income by the total number of insured members and dependents (Files and Murray 1995).

---

[19] I am grateful to my Watson Wyatt Munich colleagues Susanne Jungblut and Manuela Walkmann for this point.

FIGURE 3-4   Average Contribution Rate, Sickness Funds, 1990–1998 (as percentage of covered income)

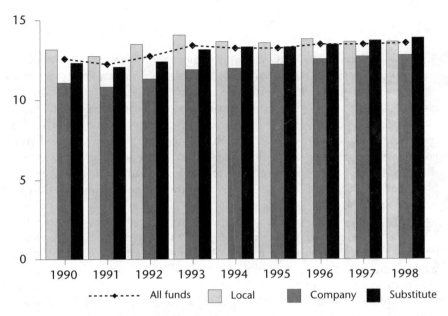

Source: Bundesministerium für Gesundheit, 1998

Note: This chart refers to the sickness funds in former western states.

This process differs from risk adjustment in the United States, for example, where income is not a factor because the insurers' income is not tied to the incomes of the insured, as in Germany (GAO 1994a).

The next set of calculations involves determining the fund's so-called standard expenditures by multiplying average cost, broken out by gender and age of a fund's membership. If a particular fund's financial strength is greater than its financial obligations to its own members, then the fund pays into the risk compensation pool, whereas if the fund's financial strength is lower than its standardized expenditures, it will be compensated from the pool (Files and Murray 1995).

The local sickness funds in the states of the former West Germany received DM 2.35 billion worth of funds in 1994—an amount equal to nearly 1.5 percent of the total spent by the sickness funds—from the risk pool fed by the wealthier funds, such as the company and substitute funds (Files and Murray 1995). As of 1997 the range of contribution rates had narrowed somewhat to between 9 and 15 percent (OECD 1997).

As Altenstetter pointed out, the equalization fund serves to obviate the need for separate insurance programs for poor and elderly individuals and so on by enabling the higher risks associated with covering such groups to be spread across the entire insurance program (Altenstetter 1998).

COMPETITION OF SORTS

January 1997 marked a watershed in the more than 100-year history of the German sickness funds system as individuals were given the freedom to chose their insurer and to switch insurers once a year. Though individuals can now choose—with certain exceptions—their sickness funds, competition is constrained by the legal requirement that the funds must offer the same comprehensive set of benefits. Funds are also prohibited from contracting with individual physicians or selected small groups; instead the funds must negotiate total physician expenditures with the regional physicians' association, though experimentation is being conducted in the form of small-scale pilot projects.

The funds will compete on their ability to keep their contribution rates low; for example, by the end of 1997 the general local funds' membership had dropped 4 percent from 1995 levels given its contribution rate was the highest among the funds (Scheil-Adlung 1998). The funds will also compete on the quality of the services they provide, as well as by offering a broader range of benefits, including disease prevention and health promotion (smoking cessation, nutrition classes, etc.) services. Indeed, because funds are subject to strict limits on advertising,[20] health promotion provides an important avenue for a fund to get its name out to potential members.

Competition is winnowing the number of sickness funds. Consolidation among funds has reduced the total number of sickness funds in the former western states from more than 1,200 in 1985 to 875 in 1995 and 443 in 1998. The number of local funds plummeted from 250 in 1992 to 12 in 1998 (Files and Murray 1995; Statistisches Bundesamt 1998).

It is hoped that through competition for members, funds will make a shift from being mere check writers (paying the bills) with a definite backseat role to more of a frontline position as mediators between patients and providers. Signs of this are already apparent; for instance, Germany's largest health insurer, Barmer Ersatzkasse, which covers 10 million people, established a monitoring department in 1996 to create disease-specific case management programs to monitor quality and costs (Marketletter 1997), and U.S. companies have provided guidance to German insurers in a wide range of managed care techniques, including utilization control,

---

[20] Advertising expenditures are limited by law to DM 6 per insured person per year (Scheil-Adlung 1998).

case management, hospital precertification, and outcomes management (Kertesz 1997).

The government continued its cost-control mission with reforms introduced in 1997, which further increased the cost burden on patients by raising copayments for pharmaceuticals to DM 9, 11, and 13 depending on the size of the prescription. The reforms also included a hike in the daily hospital copayment rate to DM 17 in the western states and DM 14 in the eastern states. In addition, coverage for certain benefits such as eyeglass frames and spa treatments was sharply curtailed. Thus reform efforts continue to focus on shifting more of the burden to patients through increased copayments, trimming back coverage of what are considered nonessential services, all with the overriding goal of maintaining universal coverage at a stable contribution rate.

CONVERGENCE

Many U.S. health policy analysts admired the German system from afar during America's national health care reform debates in the early 1990s. Germany may have returned the compliment by adopting DRG-type arrangements for hospital payments and opening up competition among the sickness funds. And there may be signs that Germany's continued march toward cost control is leading it to experiment with some of the tools of managed care.

Pilot projects, for example, have been launched that involve provider networks—a new invention in Germany. The federal association of company-based sickness funds, with 8 million members, worked with the regional association of sickness fund physicians to create a network of 150 GP practices in the Berlin area. These networked practices will be responsible for all outpatient care. Members can choose from the traditional non-networked system with free choice of physician, or the new gatekeeper-style health plan that offers discounted rates (Müller and Uedelhofen 1997). Funds are also allowed to offer rebates to enrollees with low rates of claims (Scholte and Doherty 1998).

In addition, Germany is one of the leading European nations in the use of "smart cards" for health insurance purposes—not only as identification cards to confirm individual eligibility for coverage under the sickness fund system but also to record a patient's complete medical history. It is hoped that the smart cards will enhance the coordination of care and improve the flow of information among providers (Müller and Uedelhofen 1997).

Payers and providers in the German health care system, then, deal with each other "not as individual buyers/sellers in a market, but rather as members of large organizations that engage in collective bargaining"

(Stone 1980, 75). This arrangement presents an obstacle to a central tenet of managed care; since the end of closed panels in the 1930s, insurers are forbidden by law to contract with *individual* physicians who might be willing to discount fees (Scholte and Doherty 1998). Pressure is growing, however, to allow insurance funds to negotiate costs directly with individual physicians rather than the regional associations of physicians. Moreover, pressure for change is mounting in other areas as well: Mail order pharmacies, which hold the promise of lower costs, are currently illegal in Germany, but the sickness funds are pressuring the government to relax those restrictions. But such efforts have engendered the strong resistance of individual pharmacists and the pharmaceutical industry. Managed care may have inroads into the private insurance sector in Germany, which may be more receptive to trying new ways to enhance the efficiency of care (Penn 1995).

Though Germany is unlikely to as fully embrace managed care as the United States has, certain elements will likely make their way very slowly into the German system. These will probably take the form of new ways of delivering health care services more efficiently, including strengthening the role of the sickness funds as more active purchasers and coordinators of care; methods of integrating the ambulatory and hospital care sectors to reduce costly duplication of tests and procedures and to reduce the average length of hospital stay; and training hospital professionals in hospital precertification and management techniques. Although mail order pharmacies are currently illegal, aspects of managing prescription benefits may take hold. This will gradually result in a uniquely German blend of elements of managed care within the borders of a primarily publicly financed, privately organized, universal health insurance system.

CHAPTER 4

Health Care in the Netherlands: Managed Competition Goes Dutch

The Dutch experience with health care reform provides a cautionary tale of the difficulties inherent in implementing major broad-based health care reform. The blueprint for reform drawn up in 1987 laid the framework of a reformed health care system featuring less government regulation and more market-oriented competition; the goal was to introduce regulated competition among insurers and providers to create an "internal market" for health care services, along the lines of Alain Enthoven's managed competition model. The creation of this internal market was seen as the way to enhance the efficiency of the health care system without sacrificing universal access or cost control (Jerome-Forget, White, and Wiener 1995).

Though U.S. health care reformers were once intrigued by Enthoven's managed competition as a reform approach, the Dutch actually took the idea and ran with it—or crawled with it, as it has turned out. But the Dutch reformers came at health care reform from a much different position than U.S. reformers would have: Managed competition in the Dutch context entailed introducing market-style reforms into an already heavily regulated universal health care system (Schut 1995).

The overriding goal of the reform program was to shift the responsibility for cost-control and efficiency in the health care sector from the government to the insurers, providers, and patients, through the vehicle of managed markets. Though the reform plan was initially acceptable to all political parties when released in the late 1980s, coalition governments have since changed every four years, and this has not helped move the plan along (Schut 1995). Though certain changes have been enacted over the past ten years, the "big bang" approach has fizzled and has been replaced by incremental reforms (Klein 1995a). Indeed the Dutch experience has shown that it is far easier to devise a health care reform plan than to implement one. It will be interesting to watch whether the Dutch can use managed competition to gradually transform their social insurance system into a more competitive health care system, and preserving universal access and control over costs.

This chapter begins with an overview of the Dutch health care system, followed by a description of the original health care reform program. Current progress toward reform is then discussed, as well as the major obstacles blocking progress. The chapter ends with a discussion of lessons from the Dutch experience and of whether elements of U.S. style-managed care are likely to be adopted in the Netherlands.

OVERVIEW OF THE DUTCH HEALTH CARE SYSTEM

The Dutch health care system is actually a hybrid of German social insurance and American private insurance (Janssen and van der Made 1990), and thus joins Germany in the middle range of the health care continuum. It features a blend of mandatory sickness fund-provided health insurance for the nearly two-thirds of the population that earn less than the government-set income limit of approximately $34,000 per year,[1] a separate compulsory insurance program for civil servants,[2] and private insurance for those earning incomes above the government-set ceiling. Because the income threshold is set at a lower level than in Germany, private insurance coverage casts a wider net, covering approximately one-third of the population. A separate national insurance program provides long-term care coverage for the entire population.

Beginning in the 1970s, the Dutch government administered a heavy dose of regulation over all aspects of the health care sector: prices, supply, and volume. The result was a picture of expenditure stability, particularly compared with rates of increase in other European countries, as well as in the United States. From 1980 to 1997, Dutch health care expenditures grew from 7.9 percent to 8.5 percent of GDP (OECD 1998; see Figure 4–1). At $1,975 per person, the Dutch currently spend less than half of what the United States spends on a per capita basis.

Though such enviable stability in health care expenditure rates would lead one to question why cost control would be one of the main goals of the reform program, the Dutch realized that the continued pressures of steadily advancing medical technology and an aging population would ultimately conspire to drive costs higher. The population of the Netherlands, like that of Germany, is aging at a more rapid pace than the U.S. population; more than 20 percent of the Dutch will be 65 year old or older in approximately 20 years (Table 4–1).

---

[1] The income limit for those 65 and older is approximately $20,000 per year.
[2] The civil servant insurance program covers approximately 5 percent of the population.

FIGURE 4-1   Health Care Expenditures, the Netherlands and the United States, 1971–1997 (as a percentage of GDP)

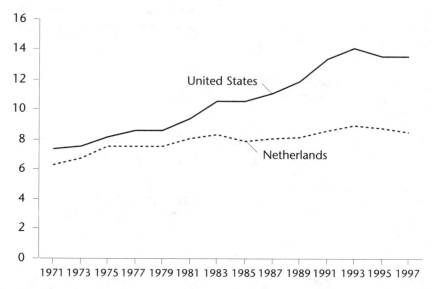

Source: OECD Health Data 98: A Comparative Analysis of 29 Countries. Paris: OECD/CREDES.

DUTCH HEALTH CARE: HISTORY AND CURRENT ORGANIZATION

Health insurance in the Netherlands, as in Germany, has its roots in medieval guilds, which set up health care organizations for their members. The system that developed was consequently one of occupation-based health insurance.

The guilds gradually gave way to other groups known broadly as sick funds, as in Germany. In 1908, for example, of the 616 sick funds, 312 were cooperatives, 230 were managed by doctors, and 74 were run for profit (de Roo 1995). By 1933 numerous health insurance groups provided voluntary coverage to 41 percent of the population (Abel-Smith 1988).

The Sickness Funds Decree of 1941 was enacted under German occupation of the Netherlands during World War II and created a health insurance program that shared many of the features of German national health insurance: mandatory participation of workers earning below a certain income limit; employer–employee contributions tied to income; and broad-based coverage of health costs related to primary care, hospital care, dental, and pharmaceutical services. Unlike in Germany, once a worker's income surpassed the income ceiling for mandatory participation, they

TABLE 4–1   Health Care in the United States and in the Netherlands

	United States	Netherlands
Life expectancy at birth, 1996	72.7 (male)	74.7 (male)
	79.4 (female)	80.4 (female)
Median age of population, 1996	35	36
Projected percentage of population over age 65		
2000	12.5	14.1
2010	13.6	16.4
2020	17.5	21.5
2030	21.9	26.0
Health care expenditures, 1997		
as percentage of GDP	13.6	8.5
per capita	$4,090	$1,975
Distribution of health care spending, 1996–1997		
Hospitals	34	53
Physicians	20	8
Pharmaceuticals	9	11
Physicians per 1,000 persons, 1994	2.6	2.6[a]
Inpatient hospital (acute) beds per 1,000 persons, 1996	4.0	11.2
Average length of stay (days), 1996	7.8	32.5
Scanners per million persons, 1993	26.9	9.0
MRIs per million persons, 1995	16.0	3.9

Sources: OECD Health Data 98: A Comparative Analysis of 29 Countries. Paris: OECD/CREDES; World Bank.
[a]1991

were compelled to leave the sickness fund system and obtain insurance through other avenues. Finally, the law held that only nonprofit sick funds could be licensed as health care insurers (de Roo 1995).

The introduction of national health insurance in the occupied Netherlands was important to the Germans for two reasons. First, they could use the sickness funds as tools to achieve their political and propaganda goals; they aimed to build support for national socialism by instituting a popular social program such as health insurance. Second, they sought to create a level playing field between German and Dutch industry because

Dutch employers would have to contribute toward the costs of their employees' insurance, as did their German counterparts (Blanpain, Delesie, and Nys 1978, 132).

After the War, the Dutch retained and subsequently built on the national health insurance program set up during the war. Though the Sickness Fund Act of 1964 required all those earning less than an annually specified income limit to become a member of a sickness fund, and therefore targeted only low to middle-income earners, the Exceptional Medical Expenses Act of 1967 introduced a mandatory universal insurance program, the Algemene Wet Bijzondere Ziektekosten (known by its initials in Dutch AWBZ) to cover the costs of long-term and catastrophic care. This separation of acute from long-term care and the low- to middle-income earners who are mandatorily covered through income-based premiums from the higher income earners who are voluntarily insured through risk-based premiums are the defining features of the Dutch health care system.

LONG-TERM CARE PROGRAM

The AWBZ is the mandatory program providing catastrophic coverage for the entire population. The program is designed to cover high-cost, high-risk services that could not be paid by individuals or adequately covered by private insurance (Ministry of Health, Welfare and Sport 1995).

The program covers care in hospitals that exceeds one year; nursing home care and other forms of institutional care; institutions for the care of the physically and mentally disabled; psychiatric institutions; and in-home nursing care.

The AWBZ is run through the sickness funds, private insurers, and insurers for civil servants. Contributions go into the Exceptional Medical Expenses Fund and health services covered under the AWBZ program are paid from this pot. The Health Insurance Funds Council oversees the insurers.

SICKNESS FUNDS COVERAGE

The nearly two-thirds of the population earning less than $34,000 per year receive coverage through a network of approximately thirty not-for-profit sickness funds, or *Ziekenfondsen,* which, as in Germany, were originally organized on a geographic basis. Insurers must cover everyone; they cannot deny coverage to individuals nor to certain employers (such as small businesses or employers in high-risk industries), and cannot exclude preexisting conditions.

Sickness funds are prohibited by law from setting up their own health care institutions or from employing physicians. Instead, they contract with health care providers. Up until 1992 each sickness fund was required to contract with "any willing provider" in its region, and the terms of the contracts between the sickness funds and the providers were negotiated at the national level between the sickness fund associations and the associations of sickness fund providers,[3] subject to approval by the Sickness Fund Council—the statutory body made up of representatives of hospitals, physicians, sickness funds, employers, employees, consumer and patient groups—that oversees the sickness fund insurance program. Since 1992 sickness funds have been able to contract with selected providers, can compete for patients on a nationwide basis, and therefore no longer have a monopoly in their region of operation (Schut 1995).

Unlike in Germany, where the level of premiums, or contributions, for sickness fund insurance is set by each sickness fund, the Dutch government sets the premium level each year. Like Germany, however, contributions are a fixed percentage of income and are not dependent on the health risk or family size of the insured.

COVERED BENEFITS

The package of benefits covered by the funds is uniform and comprehensive—covering a broad range of physician and hospital services and pharmaceuticals—and is set by the Sickness Funds Council. The council is similar to Germany's Concerted Action in that it consists of representatives of all the major health care players: physicians, hospitals, sickness funds, employers, labor unions, and the government. The council is not a government agency but does have the legal authority to regulate the sickness funds (Kirkman-Liff 1991).

Sickness funds also offer additional benefits not specified by law. More than 90 percent of individuals registered with sickness funds have such supplemental coverage for benefits not covered, or only partially covered by the compulsory program (Ministry of Health, Welfare and Sport 1995).[4]

As part of the overall reform effort in the early 1990s, the government created a Committee on Choices in Health Care to advise it on what to include or exclude from the basic package of benefits. The committee released its report in 1992, and instead of developing a detailed laundry list of benefits, the report put forth criteria for determining whether a service should be covered or not. The committee contended that each claim for services should pass four tests: whether the service is necessary to allow the individual to function in society; whether the treatment requested is

---

[3] The medical associations supported "any willing provider" regulations as a block against the return of HMO-type organizations that were prevalent in the Netherlands before the war (Schut 1995).

[4] Such supplemental benefits include dental care, home help, hearing aids, alternative medicine, and medical expenses incurred when abroad.

effective; whether the treatment is efficient; and whether the patient could pay for the service—in other words, whether it should be a matter of individual responsibility (Klein 1995b; Spanjer 1995). Dental services for adults, for example, fell into the latter category because it was determined that only preventive care for adults would be covered; coverage for physical therapy has also been scaled back.

PRIVATE INSURANCE

The Netherlands, like Germany, reserves private insurance coverage for the self-employed and high-income earners. Unlike in Germany, however, higher income earners in the Netherlands do not have the option of being covered by the sickness fund system;[5] as a result a much higher proportion of the population—three times as large as in Germany—has private insurance coverage, provided by approximately 40 private insurers. Even though this coverage is voluntary, a small share—fewer than 1 percent—of the population goes without insurance. Because most employees are mandatorily covered under the sickness fund system, only one-third of all private insurance is group insurance, similar to employer-sponsored plans in the United States (Kirkman-Liff 1991).

Private insurers determine premiums, coverage, and indemnity standards for all their enrollees except for those in high-risk groups, as discussed later. The benefits covered under private insurance tend to be similar to sickness fund benefits, but the premiums vary according to the insured's risk level, level of deductible, and hospital accommodations (OECD 1992). The majority of private insurers are members of a trade association that negotiates fees with providers (Schut 1995).

In the early 1980s the government noted that insurance premiums for certain high-risk individuals had risen very steeply and took the occasion to intervene in the private insurance market by enacting the Health Insurance Access Act of 1986. This law requires private insurers to provide standard insurance policies for high-risk individuals; the government sets the maximum premium for these policies. Though initially these standard insurance policies were available only for those with chronic conditions, in 1989 the government extended the protection to all individuals over age 65.

---

[5] Voluntary sickness fund insurance was eliminated in 1986 (OECD 1992). Many individuals who are forced to switch to private insurance when their income level exceeds the limit choose to be insured by the not-for-profit subsidiary insurance company tied to their former sickness fund (Saltman and Figueras 1998). This is not surprising given people's familiarity with the way the insurer does business, that all their information is already in the insurer's system, and that it is not unusual for the employer to have a group contract with the sickness fund subsidiary. I am grateful to my Watson Wyatt Amsterdam colleague Ton Pouwels for this information.

The price of the standard policy is less than the actual expenditures, and the policies are subsidized by a risk pool into which all privately insured patients pay. Since the extension of the standard insurance requirement for all those over age 65, 40 percent of private health insurance now falls within the mandatory risk pool (OECD 1992; Schut 1995).

HEALTH CARE FINANCING

Sickness fund insurance is financed by employer–employee-paid, income-based premiums. Premiums for sickness fund coverage amounted to slightly more than 7 percent of covered income in 1998. Unlike in Germany, where contributions are split evenly between employers and employees, Dutch employers contribute the lion's share of premiums, paying 5.85 percent to the employee's 1.55 percent of covered income. In addition to their share of the premiums, all insured adults pay a flat-rate premium of approximately $175 per year to their sickness funds. Employers contribute the same amount to the cost of private insurance for their high-income employees as they do for the employees covered under sickness fund-administered insurance plans.

The national catastrophic medical plan is also financed by income-related premiums that amounted to 10.25 percent of an employee's salary in 1999. Employers do not contribute directly to the AWBZ, but do so indirectly through additional wages that partially compensate for the employee contribution to the long-term care program (Spencer and Associates 1998).

In terms of overall health care financing, the largest share of health care revenues are generated through the income-based premiums collected by the sickness funds, with the next largest share represented by the long-term and catastrophic care program (Figure 4–2).

HEALTH CARE DELIVERY

The health care delivery system of the Netherlands is predominantly private, though the government is never far away.

PHYSICIANS

There were 2.6 physicians per 1,000 population in the Netherlands as of 1991.[6] Unlike in Germany, the Dutch government regulates the number of medical students through a lottery system, so the number of general physi-

---

[6] The most recent year for which such statistics are available is 1991.

FIGURE 4-2   Dutch Health Care Financing, 1996, by Source of Funds
(in percentages)

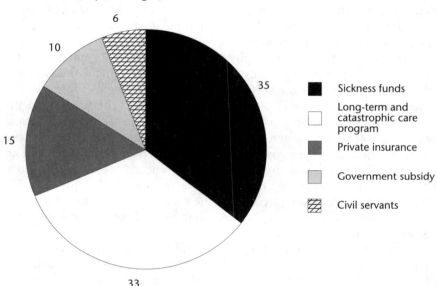

Legend:
- Sickness funds
- Long-term and catastrophic care program
- Private insurance
- Government subsidy
- Civil servants

Source: "Health Care in the Netherlands 1996." Royal Netherlands Embassy (www.netherlands-embassy.org)

cians and specialists can ultimately be controlled. As in Germany, there is a sharp separation between general practitioners (GPs) and specialists. Approximately three quarters of all specialists are private contractors who are in hospital-based partnerships with an average of six specialists. The remaining one quarter of all specialists are employed primarily by university hospitals (Schut 1995).

GPs play a key role as the gatekeepers that control access to specialists and hospitals. Dutch GPs have a "strong family practice orientation with a tradition of comprehensive care and home visits" (Mullan 1998, 123). Every sickness fund-insured individual must register with a GP who has a contract with their sickness fund. In contrast, privately insured patients have free choice of GP. GPs are independent contractors, and most are in solo practices (with an average of approximately 2,000 patients), although proposed reforms include incentives to form more group practices (Mullan 1998; Schut 1995).

Physician reimbursement methods in the Netherlands vary, depending on whether the physician is a GP or a specialist and whether the physician is treating a sickness fund or privately insured patient. GPs are paid on a fee-for-service basis for private insurance patients, but are paid on a capitation (per person) basis for patients enrolled in sickness funds. Most physicians treat both sickness-fund insured patients and privately insured patients. Almost all specialists are paid on a fee-for-service basis for patients under both the private and sickness fund plans (Kirkman-Liff 1991).

More than 90 percent of all GPs belong to a national association representing physicians in negotiations with both the sickness funds and private insurers to determine physician fee levels and capitation rates (Kirkman-Liff 1989). Physician payment levels for general practitioners contracting with sickness funds are calculated according to a formula that takes into account three factors: the "norm income," the "norm patient-list size," and the "norm practice costs" for physicians. The norm income is not an average or median income but an income range negotiated between physicians and the government. The norm patient-list size is not an average or median size either, but rather a standard, negotiated practice size (for example, the norm practice size was set at 2,350 patients in 1988). The norm practice cost figure reflects the costs of all elements of a physician's practice, including office space, labor costs of medical and office assistants, and medical equipment.[7]

The sum of the norm income figure and the norm practice cost figure is then divided by the norm practice size to arrive at a monthly capitation rate. This is the per-person rate that the sickness fund will pay the general practitioner (Kirkman-Liff 1989). The capitation payment is designed so that the annual income of a GP with a standard-sized practice is roughly comparable to that of a highly ranked government official (Schut 1995).

General practitioners who contract with private insurers, on the other hand, are paid according to a fee schedule. The schedule has a fixed price for services such as routine office visits, telephone consultations, and home visits.

Independent specialists belong to the National Association of Specialists, which is charged with negotiating their fee schedule. Specialists are paid on a fee-for-service basis according to separate fee schedules, one for sickness fund-insured patients and one for privately insured patients. The latter tends to have fees nearly twice as high as the sickness fund fee schedule (Schut 1995).

At one time the sickness funds attempted to monitor specialists' incomes. The total amount billed by each specialist was to be added up every year and compared against the norm income for specialists. Any specialist who had exceeded the norm income was to pay back part of the excess. The practice was intended to discourage specialists from over-servicing to increase their incomes (Kirkman-Liff 1989). Though the specialists agreed on the arrangement with the sickness funds, ultimately it fell to the govern-

---

[7] The cost of cars and gasoline is also factored in, as Dutch physicians are expected to make house calls.

ment to enforce the agreement and ensure the specialists did indeed reimburse the funds for any excess beyond the limit. The expenditure targets were exceeded in 1990 and 1991, for example, and as a result the government reduced all specialists' fees in 1993 to recoup the excess (Schut 1995).

The government has indicated that it intends to make all specialists salaried employees of the hospital for which they work. Approximately half of all specialists are on salary, whereas the rest are still paid on a fee-for-service basis, with their fees tied to the budget negotiated between the insurers, the hospital, and its specialists (Kirkman-Liff 1996).

HOSPITALS

Private for-profit hospitals are prohibited in the Netherlands; 85 percent of all hospitals are private not-for-profit institutions and the remainder are public hospitals (OECD 1992). Excess hospital capacity is evident in the large number of hospital beds—11.2 per 1,000 population—nearly three times the U.S. level. At 32.5 days, the Dutch average length of hospital stay also exceeds that of all other nations in this study, except Japan.

Though hospitals are mainly private independent institutions, they are heavily regulated by the government, with limits on capital expenditures imposed in 1975 and global budgeting in 1983. The central government limits hospital supply and technology purchases through its licensing authority; hospitals need the government's permission to expand facilities or purchase new medical technologies (Jonssen 1990; Lapre 1988). The 1983 law requires hospitals to operate within the confines of a predetermined budget that is negotiated with the sickness funds and private insurers according to guidelines set by the Central Office on Health Care Prices (Schut 1995). The government also sets guidelines on the maximum annual growth of labor costs, which are used in collective negotiations between representatives of the hospital and the labor unions over nonmedical hospital employees' wages (OECD 1992).

HEALTH CARE REFORM IN THE NETHERLANDS

Following a severe recession in the 1970s, the Dutch turned to heavy government intervention to control costs in the health care sector. Yet the strong belief in a large role for government in society that predominated in the 1970s gradually gave way to the perception that heavy government regulation was a hindrance rather than a help (Schut 1995). In 1982 the Dutch government introduced an economy-wide privatization program, which triggered an overall reassessment of the role of government in the health care sector. The Health Care Prices Act of 1982 created the Central

Office on Health Care Prices, made up of representatives of providers, insurers, and the government—an attempt to create a more balanced approach than relying solely on government to set health care prices and fees.

The reassessment of government's role in the health care sector crystallized in 1987 with the publication of the report of the Committee on the Structure and Financing of the Health Care System. Known as the Dekker Committee after its chair Dr. W. Dekker, former CEO of Dutch electronics giant Philips, the committee issued a report titled "Willingness to Change," which spelled out specific plans for the complete restructuring of the Dutch health care system (Janssen and van der Made 1990; Lapre 1988; Ministry of Welfare, Health and Cultural Affairs, 1988).

The Dekker Committee concluded that the increased government involvement in the health care sector introduced in the mid-1970s did not address the underlying weaknesses in the system, most notably the absence of incentives for improved efficiency and cost control. Cost-consciousness on the part of patients was nonexistent because they were fully covered for health care services. Insurers were fully reimbursed for their expenditures; moreover, they were required to enter into contracts with any provider in their region, and thus served mainly as check writers rather than prudent purchasers and managers of health care services (van de Ven and Schut 1995). In addition, the committee found the need for better coordination of health services, including the substitution of more cost-effective treatments, such as the use of ambulatory care rather than inpatient care wherever possible.

The committee's proposals had a decidedly market flair: The emphasis would be shifted from government regulation to market regulation, and competitive forces would be introduced to make the system more efficient. Health care consumers, providers, and payers would be expected to increase their responsibility for health care cost control. The committee explicitly stated, however, that increased competition would not come at the expense of health care quality and equity (Ministry of Welfare, Health and Cultural Affairs 1988).

The reforms were to create what one analyst characterized as a "social system in a market-oriented setting" (van Etten 1990). The government would let market forces work their magic while keeping a watchful eye over the system. Government regulation would not be replaced by the market; it would exist in a different form—government reregulation rather than deregulation (van de Van and Schut 1995).

The committee determined that it was necessary to eliminate the public–private system that had developed, given that the public plans wound up covering the higher risk individuals, with the private plans covering the lower risk individuals. The reform program aimed to eliminate the distinction between public and private by replacing the existing four-part system with a single health insurance program for the entire population regardless of income level.

This new compulsory public plan would be established to cover the basic and catastrophic health expenses of the entire population, with the basic benefits to be covered under the program set by law. Optional supplemental insurance would be available to cover such services as certain prescription drugs, private hospital rooms, cosmetic surgery, and so on.

All Dutch residents would continue to pay income-based premiums set by the government. These premiums would cover 75 percent of the program's cost, and the remaining 25 percent would come from a flat-rate premium (not based on income). Insurers would not be able to charge different premium rates, but the flat-rate premiums, which were designed to encourage competition between the sickness fund and private insurance companies, could vary. Insurers that negotiated the most cost-effective arrangements with providers would be able to offer lower flat-rate premium rates, and would therefore attract the most patients. The introduction of flat-rate premiums was also based on the assumption that the insured would become more aware of the cost of health care if they had to bear some of the burden themselves (Ministry of Welfare, Health and Cultural Affairs 1989).

Although the flat-rate premiums would be paid to the insurers directly, the income-based premiums would be collected through standard tax collection channels and put into one central fund, which would act as the system's paymaster, making capitated allocations to insurers based on the risk composition of the insured population. In other words, the fund would collect income-related premiums and then make payments to competing insurers based on the risk status of their members. Insurers that covered a large number of high-risk individuals would receive compensation from the central fund (Greenberg 1990; Lapre 1988).

The government would be involved in defining the basic package of benefits to be covered by the new insurance program, set the maximum premium insurers could charge, control hospital capacity, and regulate the competition among insurers to ensure that universal access and equity were not threatened.

A REFORM PLAN BY ANY OTHER NAME

The governing center-right coalition was replaced with a center-left governing coalition in 1990. The new government modified the Dekker Plan to expand its scope of coverage. The new plan, named Plan Simons,[8] was, like its predecessor, designed to cover the basic and catastrophic health

---

[8] Named after Hans Simons, the Secretary of State for Health at the time.

expenses of the entire Dutch population. The program's comprehensive benefits were expected to cover 96 percent of total health care expenditures, with supplemental insurance available to cover remaining expenditures. Plan Simons changed the financing ratio of income-related and flat-rate premiums from 75 : 25 to 82 : 18.

As under the Dekker Plan, insurers were to compete to provide basic health benefits, negotiating prices with competing health care providers. Maximum provider fees would still be regulated by the government, but insurers could contract with selected providers for lower rates, and the flat-rate premium would vary by insurer. The central fund would still control the lion's share of the payment to insurers (Jerome-Forget, White, and Wiener 1995). Nevertheless the Simons Plan significantly toned down the Dekker reforms' emphases on market forces.

The plan was to use the AWBZ as the vehicle for the basic insurance program for all, and to that end the government began transferring certain services from coverage under sickness fund and private insurance programs to the AWBZ. As of 1992, for example, coverage for pharmaceuticals, medical equipment, and rehabilitative services were transferred to the AWBZ.

This transfer of benefits turned out to be the health reform program's undoing. As benefits were transferred to the AWBZ program from sickness fund and private insurance, income-related contributions replaced the risk-related premiums previously charged for those benefits. This did not sit well with middle to higher income earners (Schut 1995).

REFORM'S FORWARD (AND BACKWARD) MOVEMENT

A change in government in 1994 sealed the fate of health care reform. The new government decided that the AWBZ was to be kept in its original form as the program for catastrophic care, separate from the competitive program for basic insurance (van Barneveld et al. 1995). The previously mentioned services were transferred back to coverage under sickness fund and private insurance plans in 1996.

The new government shifted the emphasis away from market competition and back toward government regulation, most notably in measures designed to control costs in the pharmaceutical sector. Although the Dutch do not use pharmaceuticals as heavily as, for example, the Germans or Japanese, the government determined that the price of pharmaceuticals was approximately 20 to 25 percent higher than elsewhere in Europe. The Netherlands uses a negative list, which is to say drugs not included on the list are not reimbursable. The Medicine Pricing Act of 1996 set maximum prices for drugs that represent the average of the price of the drug in Belgium, France, Germany, and the United Kingdom. The average price is the maximum price above which the patient will not be reimbursed. Finally, a requirement mandating that consumers pay 20 percent of pharmaceuticals was introduced in 1997 (Royal Embassy of the Netherlands 1997; Scheil-Adlung 1998).

OUTLOOK FOR THE FUTURE

As the Dutch begin their second decade of experience in health care reform, it is not clear where the reforms will go. A new labour-led governing coalition was formed in July 1998. The one step forward-two steps back dance over the past decade has left the impression that a long-term vision is seriously lacking.

Despite the fact that reform has been characterized by a series of fits and starts, there are clear signs of change: The sickness funds, which for half a century had received full reimbursement for their medical expenditures and therefore had no incentive to negotiate on price and quality with providers, now have an incentive to do so given that they are paid a capitated amount from the central fund. They are gradually making the transformation from "administrative bodies into risk-bearing, consumer-oriented organizations" (van de Ven and Schut 1995, 104), charged with buying cost-effective care for their members. Indeed, with the advent of selective contracting, the sickness funds are no longer under obligation to contract with any provider in their region. Sickness funds and private insurers are free to negotiate discounted fees, which up until 1992 had been illegal. Other steps to the market include the fact that sickness funds can now operate on a nationwide basis; patients can choose among sickness funds at least every two years; and sickness funds can compete on quality, range of services, and responsiveness to patients (van de Ven and Schut 1995).

Overall, the government had set a target annual growth rate for health care spending of 1.3 percent, but in the past two years, growth rates have been in the range of 4 percent. The government is now looking at raising the target growth rate to 2.6 percent.

One pressing problem that the government must face is that budgets for specialized services have led to waiting times of several months—for example, for coronary bypass surgery, laser treatments for retinal bleeding—with much longer waiting times for elective surgery. Employers are affected by waiting lists, because as of 1996 the financial responsibility for cash sickness benefits was shifted from the social security program to employers. Employers are now required to pay cash sickness benefits for an employee's first fifty-two weeks of absence from work. If the employee has to wait for hospital care, thereby delaying treatment, recovery, and subsequent return to work, the employer feels the direct impact. This combined with the fact that employers pay a large share of an employee's health care premium will ensure that employers will become more actively involved in the management of health care services and costs (*IBIS Review* 1997).

The government for its part has sought to reduce the waiting lists by infusing more cash into the system. This entailed an additional $24 million in 1997 and $100 million in 1998 (Spencer and Associates 1998).

CHANGING ROLES IN THE DUTCH HEALTH CARE SECTOR

The Dutch experience in some ways resembles that of Germany: Health care reform is not a one-shot deal, but rather a constantly evolving process that involves periodic retooling. The Dutch were overly optimistic on the timetable for reform, having expected to complete their comprehensive reform program in a relatively brief period of five years. Moreover, they underestimated the technical complexity involved in setting an appropriately refined risk-adjusted capitation payment.

Indeed, one of the primary lessons from the Dutch experience is that the successful creation of a well-functioning competitive market for health insurance that does not feature cream-skimming—the selection of preferred risks—by the insurers is predicated on sufficiently refined risk-adjusted capitation payments. This is critical in the Dutch system because the bulk of the insurers' medical expenditures are to be covered by the risk-adjusted capitation payment from the central fund.

The capitation formula used in the Dutch system initially adjusted only for the two factors of age and gender of the insured. Yet this was seen to be insufficient; the sickness funds in Amsterdam, for example, had higher than average costs because of a high incidence of AIDS patients and those addicted to drugs as well as low-income individuals who tended to have higher health care expenditures. The existing formula was not adequate to compensate for these different health risks. By 1995 geographic location and disability were added to the formula (Schut 1995; van de Ven and Schut 1995).

Research indicates in fact that variables such as age and gender can explain only a very small portion of the variation in individual health care expenditures. A host of other factors are needed to make the risk-adjustment formula more refined and thus more able to predict the health care costs of a given individual, ranging from employment status, family size, and socioeconomic status to chronic conditions, physical impairments, and self-rated general health status. Adding together all these factors can greatly enhance the predictive power of the formula (Hamilton 1995). Until the government settles on the right risk-adjusted capitation payment formula, the likelihood of cream skimming by insurers will continue to exist, and the sickness funds will not be able to become the risk-bearing enterprises envisioned by the reform (van de Ven and Schut 1995).

The Dutch experience also points to the difficulties involved in striking a working balance between governmental regulation and competitive insurance markets. The Dutch have taken significant, if not giant, steps away from governmental control over the health care sector that predominated during the 1970s. The government has retained its influential presence in the health care system even as changes are made to make the system more competitive and more reliant on market forces. Indeed, government regulation has not been replaced by the competitive forces—instead it has changed its stripes from direct control over health care prices, volume, and supply to monitoring health outcomes. The state is to set overall objectives and regulate the main health care actors to ensure objectives are met. The goal is to get the state to "row less and steer more" (Osborne and Gaebler, quoted in Saltman and Figueras 1998).

The government reserves the right to fix the income-related component of the premiums for basic insurance and legislate the scope of basic insurance coverage, while allowing insurers to compete with one another for patients. Thus in the Netherlands, as in Germany, even though competitive market forces are being introduced into the health care system, the government maintains an important regulatory role.

CONVERGENCE

One common element of managed care, the primacy of primary care and reliance on gatekeepers, is well-established in the Netherlands. Indeed the Dutch tradition of GP-as-gatekeeper has provided what health expert Chris Ham has called "a money-saving first-stop shop for quality care" (Ham 1998). Dutch GPs have long lived within a managed care-style capitated payment system.

GPs will be relied on to play an even more active role in the reforming system, going beyond gatekeeper to "coordinator or professional personal guide to the health care system," ensuring that the system functions at its maximum level of efficiency (Mullan 1998, 123). And one should not underestimate the impact of gatekeeping on overall management of health care services (Saltman and Figueras 1998). Consider that the number of physician contacts per person in gatekeeper-oriented Dutch and British systems were more than twice as high in the Japanese system, where gatekeeping is nonexistent (Figure 4–3).

In the pharmaceutical sector, the Dutch have been able to do what Germany has not: Take a step toward managed care with the launch of mail-order pharmacies. In late 1996 Caremark International, one of the leading U.S. Pharmacy Benefit Management (PBM) companies, set up a PBM program in the Netherlands, which provides mail-order pharmacy service to the more than one million people insured by Holland's largest private health insurance company, Zilveren Kruis (Silver Cross; Edlin 1997). The introduction of mail-order pharmacies received a decidedly less-than-

FIGURE 4-3   Keeping the Gate: Physician Consultations per Person, 1995–1996

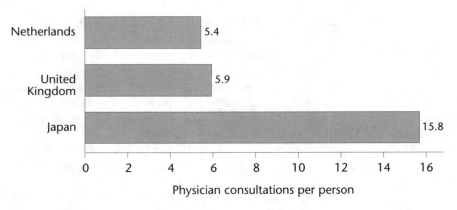

Source: OECD Health Data 98: A Comparative Analysis of 29 Countries. Paris: OECD/CREDES.

warm welcome from Dutch pharmacists and drug wholesalers who worked hard to block their entrance into the Dutch system. The outlook for such mail-order pharmacies in the Netherlands is therefore unclear.

The Dutch, like the Germans, are also experimenting with data-embedded "smart cards" that hold patient medical information so that physicians and pharmacists can coordinate treatment and avoid adverse drug interactions. The use of such smart cards is pervasive in the private insurance sector, where insurers use the cards to identify the patient and his or her level of coverage (Life Insurance International 1997).

These and other changes indicate that the Dutch health care system continues to evolve one decade after the initial reform blueprint was proposed, a blueprint of a system of regulated competition among insurers, modeled to a significant degree on American ideas. The United Kingdom has also turned to those same American concepts, having enacted significant reforms of the National Health Service based on Enthoven's concepts of managed competition (see Chapter 7).

Students of health care policy will be interested to see how the Netherlands navigates the choppy waters of health care reform and what the effect will be on equity and effectiveness in that health care system. If the Dutch can successfully blend competitive markets and government regulation, they may master the health care dilemma many other nations are facing.

CHAPTER 5

Made in Japan:
Universal Health Insurance

Japan's health care system presents a "tantalizing puzzle" (Ikegami and Campbell 1995, 1,295) of positive and negative aspects of health care systems. The Japanese system is complex yet straightforward, fragmented yet egalitarian, predominantly private yet subject to strict governmental regulation, provides universal coverage for far less money than the United States devotes to health care and yields positive health outcomes yet suffers from significant quality problems.

This chapter begins with an overview of Japanese health care, followed by a section that traces the roots of Japan's complex health care system and identifies the cultural influences that have shaped its development. Subsequent sections detail the organization and financing of health care in Japan, areas for reform, as well as potential lessons for the United States.

Japan is to Asia what Germany was to Europe: the first nation to introduce a comprehensive social insurance program. The Japanese turned to Bismarck's program as a model for their own version of social insurance, which features universal coverage attained through a mandate on all residents to join a health insurance plan, either through place of employment or residence, and a mandate on all companies employing five or more workers to contribute to a health plan for their employees. The system is financed through employer–employee contributions, which are based on income, combined with government subsidies for certain groups. Though there are multiple payers and a predominantly private delivery system, as in the U.S. health care system, the government ensures that all plans offer a comprehensive set of uniform benefits and has the power to set the fees for all covered services through a nationwide, uniform fee schedule that governs all payments to all payers. This public–private mix locates Japan in the middle of the health care continuum.

THE JAPANESE ADVANTAGE

The United States turned its attention to the Japanese health care system during the 1980s, when rapidly escalating U.S. health care costs led U.S.

executives—particularly those in the auto industry—to frequently be-moan what they considered to be Japan's unfair advantage: that U.S. car makers' health care costs were as high as "$3,500 a year per employee [whereas] the Japanese are paying virtually nothing" (*Wall Street Journal* 1990). Although this statement is not entirely accurate—Japanese firms do contribute to their employees' health care costs by paying part of the em-ployee's premium as well as through corporate tax revenues to finance health programs for the elderly—it reflected a commonly held belief that high U.S. health care costs put American companies at a disadvantage when competing with Japanese firms. Though health care expenses alone do not determine whether a company is competitive or not, they do con-stitute a significant portion of a company's total labor costs (Maher 1990; Mitchell 1990; Reinhardt 1989, 1990; Schramm 1990).

U.S. attention has also focused on the relative parsimony[1] of the Japanese health care system: Whereas U.S. and Japanese health care costs experienced similar rates of increase throughout the 1970s, Japan man-aged to keep a tighter rein on health care expenditures in the 1980s than did the United States (Figure 5–1). This changed in the 1990s, however, as health care costs increased in Japan significantly, from 6 percent of GDP in 1990 to slightly more than 7 percent of GDP in 1997.

Japan devotes far fewer financial resources to health care than the United States, while providing health insurance coverage for its entire population. Universal coverage is a relatively recent achievement; Japan has successfully made the transition from a nation considered to be a "welfare laggard" to a nation with a system of universal health insurance with highly beneficial health outcomes (Steslicke 1982). Japan leads the world in terms of life expectancy at birth (76.4 years for men and 82.8 years for women)—an impressive achievement given that four decades ago life expectancy rates in Japan were only 50 years for men and 53.9 years for women.

Average life expectancy rates at older ages have also improved dra-matically. In 1965 average life expectancy at age 65 was 11.9 years for men and 14.6 years for females. As of 1995, 65-year-old Japanese men could

---

[1] Many analysts question whether Japan's costs are as low as they seem. Japanese government health figures are lower than those compiled by the OECD because they do not include all health care services, in particular medical research and education, grants to public hospitals, over-the-counter drugs, preventive health care services, or gifts—"tips"—to physicians. The OECD has es-timated total health care costs using a standardized format for each country, and their figures do account for many of the services not included in the official Japanese government figures. Ana-lysts have estimated that accounting for the under-the-table payments to physicians would raise the OECD figure by less than 5 percent (Ikegami and Campbell 1995; Katsumata 1996). Ikegami and Campbell thus concluded that the low rates of Japanese health care spending are truly low and not merely "an artifact of differences in statistical compilation methods" (Ikegami and Camp-bell 1995, 1,295).

FIGURE 5-1   Japanese and United States Health Care Expenditures, 1971–1997
            (as a percentage of GDP)

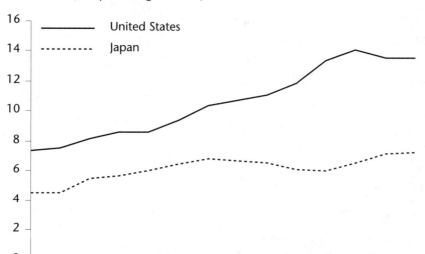

Source: *OECD Health Data 98: A Comparative Analysis of 29 Countries.* Paris: OECD/CREDES.

expect to live another 16.5 years, and women another 20.9 years (Matsunaga 1997). Japan also boasts infant mortality rates that are among the world's lowest. It would seem that Japan has achieved a "health miracle" comparable to its success in the economic and business spheres (Steslicke 1989, 104).

It is important to note that the relationship between such broad health care outcome measures and the particular structure of the health care system is unclear. The health care system is only one of myriad factors that contribute to a nation's health outcomes. Indeed, other factors such as diet, nutrition, health prevention, income and education levels of the population, and prevalence of diseases such as Acquired Immune Deficiency Syndrome (AIDS), as well as levels of alcohol and substance abuse and violent crime, very likely have more to do with health outcomes than the particulars of the health care system.

Certainly, the cultural, social, and political differences between Japan and the United States far outweigh the similarities and serve as limiting factors on the applicability of the Japanese health care system as a model for U.S. health care reform. Differences in population sizes and ethnic makeup are significant, and wide disparities in income and education levels that exist in the United States are negligible in Japan. Other factors include the

TABLE 5–1   Health Care in the United States and Japan

	United States	Japan
Life expectancy at birth, 1995	72.7 (male) 79.4 (female)	77.0 (male) 83.6 (female)
Median age of population, 1996	35	40
Projected percentage of population age 65 or older		
2000	12.5	17.2
2010	13.6	22.0
2020	17.5	26.9
Health care expenditures, 1996		
as % GDP	13.6	7.3
per capita	$4,090	$1,741
Distribution of health care spending, 1996–1997 (as percent of total spending)		
Hospitals	34	29[a]
Physicians	20	34
Drugs	8	20
Physicians per 1,000 persons, 1996	2.6	1.8
Inpatient hospital beds per 1,000 persons, 1996	4.0	16.2[a]
Average length of stay (days), 1995	7.8	45.5[b]
% of population admitted	12.4	8.9[a]
Number of surgical operations per 1,000 persons[c]	91	22
Scanners per million persons	26.9 (1993)	69.7 (1996)
MRIs per million persons	16.0 (1995)	18.8 (1996)

Sources: OECD Health Data 98: A Comparative Analysis of 29 Countries. Paris: OECD/CREDES; World Bank; National Institute of Population and Social Security Research, Ministry of Health and Welfare of Japan.

[a] 1994 data.
[b] Includes long-term stay patients. Note: The ALOS for general hospitals in Japan is 33.7 days. I am grateful to Mr. Kazuhito Ihara, Director, Health and Welfare Department, JETRO for this information.
[c] From 1986 American Hospital Association Annual Survey data and Ministry of Health and Welfare patient survey, cited in Ikegami 1991.

fact that the United States has an extremely litigious society in which the threat of malpractice suits drives defensive medicine, whereas malpractice suits are relatively rare in Japan. And though the aging of the population demands U.S. attention, it pales in comparison to the demographic tsunami that will hit Japan in a few years (Table 5–1). Indeed, demographics will set the future course of the Japanese health care system, because in the short span of two decades, the share of the Japanese population over age 65 will soar from 17 percent in 2000 to nearly 27 percent in 2020.[2]

The math gets scary when one considers that approximately one-third of Japan's total health care bill is already spent on services for the elderly, who currently represent less than 17 percent of the population (Figure 5–2). Not only do the elderly tend to consume greater amounts of health care services, but given that the Japanese health care system is financed mainly through premiums tied to wages, the aging of the population will have a particularly significant impact as fewer workers are called on to fund the increasing cost of health care.

The cost pressures brought on by a rapidly aging population are amplified by Japan's current economic malaise. The bloom is off the rose of Japan's vaunted economic miracle as the high-powered engine of Japan Inc. began to sputter in the early 1990s and has spent the last years of the 1990s mired in recession. Just as system-wide reform is necessary to get Japan's financial and economic house in order, many changes need to be made within the health care arena as well. Though health care spending as a percentage of GDP is well below U.S. levels, as noted earlier, costs are rising significantly, and given the demographics they will continue to do so. Japan recently administered a dose of harsh medicine by raising the financial burden borne by patients by doubling out-of-pocket payments and increasing premiums, and targeted the pharmaceutical industry for cost-control measures by slicing the reimbursement prices of drugs.

Though the differences between the two nations are important, Japan's experience in providing universal coverage and controlling costs, as well as the ways in which it manages health care services for its rapidly aging population, offer lessons the United States cannot afford to ignore.

CONFLUENCE OF EAST AND WEST

It is often noted that the Japanese, located at the confluence of East and West, exhibit a remarkable ability to absorb the best of other systems and tailor them to their own environment (Hashimoto 1984, 335). This is certainly true in the health care domain; the major influences on the development of the Japanese health care system include Chinese, Dutch, and German medicine. Traditional Chinese medicine made its debut in Japan

---

[2] Population aging has occurred at a particularly rapid pace in Japan. The proportion of the Japanese population age 65 or older doubled from 7 to 14 percent over the span of slightly more than two decades (1970–1994). The same expansion took 46 years in the United Kingdom and 42 in Germany, and is expected to take 69 years in the United States (Morishita 1998).

FIGURE 5-2   Health Care Expenditures in Japan, 1995 (in percentages)

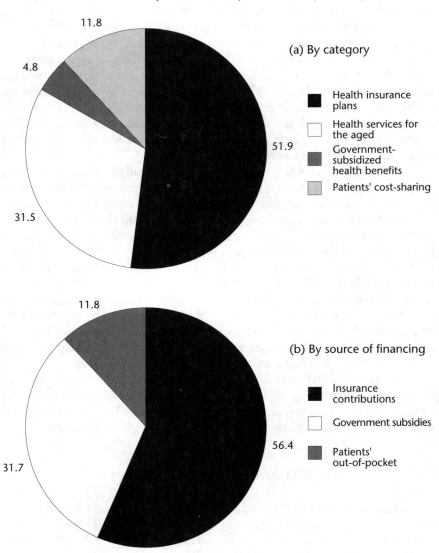

(a) By category

■ Health insurance plans

□ Health services for the aged

▨ Government-subsidized health benefits

▨ Patients' cost-sharing

(b) By source of financing

■ Insurance contributions

□ Government subsidies

▨ Patients' out-of-pocket

Source: Ministry of Health and Welfare, Japan

during the sixth century A.D. and featured treatment based primarily on the use of acupuncture and herbal medicines. The Chinese influence is still evident today, as we will see, in Japan's relatively heavy reliance on prescription drugs for treatment and in the lack of a formal separation between pharmacist and physician (Ikegami and Campbell 1995).

It was a thousand years after the influence of the Chinese before Japan felt the influence of Western medical practices through contact with Portuguese missionary programs. But in the early 1600s Japan essentially closed its borders and underwent an extended isolationist period that lasted until the mid-1800s. Chinese and Dutch traders were exempt from the ban on foreigners, however, and it was through this route that Japan was introduced to Dutch medical care practices, which had a profound impact on the shape of Japan's health care system (Iglehart 1988a).

Japan was torn by a civil war in 1867, known as the Meiji Restoration, which witnessed the elimination of the feudal system by "an alliance of powerful landowners, young samurai and mercantile capitalists." The subsequent period—the Meiji Era (1868 to 1912)—was one of the more important periods in the evolution of Japanese society, as an industrialized nation was born within the relatively short span of a few decades (Hashimoto 1984, 336).

Japan became increasingly open to Western influences during this period, as the nation's leaders looked to other countries for ideas that were compatible with their drive toward modernization. Japanese leaders believed that Japan's industrialization was perfectly timed because Japan could not only learn from mistakes already made by Western industrialized nations but would also be forewarned of potential problems related to industrialization (Steslicke 1982). The major influences during this period include the British Navy and Merchant Marines, the Prussian Army, and even American business.

Japan's leaders were particularly attracted to Germany's health care system, which was considered to be the best in Europe at that time (Hashimoto 1984). Even the underlying political and economic conditions in Japan in the early twentieth century resembled those in Germany in the mid-1800s: The forces of industrialization and the development of organized labor groups had stirred up public demands for social welfare programs. In the words of historian Kenneth Pyle, the Japanese version of German social policy was based on the concept of "a monarch and a neutral bureaucracy standing above narrow class interests, regulating economic conditions, reconciling opposing social forces, and seeking to advance the interests of the whole by intervening in the economy to protect and integrate the lower classes into the nation" (Steslicke 1982, 202).

The Japanese government of this era, similar to that of Bismarck's Germany, wanted to ensure a steady supply of healthy workers to drive economic growth as well as to maintain control over the workers. The Bis-marckian mixture of repression and social legislation was an appropriate means to this end and remained a primary influence on the development of Japanese health care through the end of World War II (Hashimoto 1984; Steslicke 1982). The use of a national system of health insurance as a means of quelling nascent socialist movements in Germany and Japan stands in stark contrast to U.S. experience, wherein national health insur-ance, dubbed "socialized medicine," is viewed as part of a broader social-ist agenda (Ikegami 1991).

Though Japan relied on the German model in constructing its na-tionwide system of health insurance, one important distinction bears pointing out. Japan does not allow anyone to opt out of the mandated health insurance system to purchase private insurance for benefits covered by the national health insurance program. That everyone is in the same health care boat, so to speak, has important implications for the system's financing and cost control.

LEGISLATING HEALTH INSURANCE COVERAGE

The cornerstone of the present-day Japanese health insurance system was laid by the enactment of the Health Insurance Law of 1922, which was de-signed to provide health insurance coverage to such major occupational groups as factory workers and miners. Excluded from the law were em-ployers with fewer than five workers, self-employed individuals such as agricultural workers, and those involved in fishing and forestry (Steslicke 1982). This new employment-based health insurance law created two gen-eral categories of insurers. Companies with more than 700 employees were to form health insurance societies that would provide medical facil-ities for employees or cover the cost of care at a medical facility. The other insurer was to be the government; it would manage health insurance pro-grams for employees of smaller firms not covered by insurance societies (Steslicke 1982).

The progression toward codification of social policy continued with the enactment of the National Health Insurance Law in 1938. This law re-quired local governments to extend health insurance coverage to those not covered by the 1922 law, such as individuals involved in farming, fishing, and forestry. Driven by simultaneous desires to foster economic growth and to prevent a widening income gap from causing social instability, the Japanese government revised the 1938 law in 1958 with the aim of mak-ing health insurance coverage universal (Steslicke 1982).

The 1958 revision of the law was designed to provide insurance cov-erage to those not covered by previous legislation—approximately 30 per-

cent of the population (Steslicke 1989). The new law was based on residence, whereas previous laws were organized around employment. Every
jurisdiction—city, town, or village—was required to implement a health
insurance program by 1961.

Thus the health insurance system in Japan, as in Germany, developed
gradually, incorporating larger portions of the population over time. Rather
than create an entirely new system, the government built on the existing
system and subsequently imposed a nationwide set of regulations to govern the system. By the early 1960s, virtually the entire population was covered by a health insurance plan—either one offered by employers or one
administered by local governments or trade associations.

ORGANIZED COMPLEXITY

The Japanese system features multiple insurers in a fragmented network
of programs and plans. Though complex, the system is straightforward in
that every Japanese resident must enroll in a health insurance plan, either
through their employer or their local government or trade association. All
companies with five or more employees must contribute toward the cost
of their employees' health care premiums.

The health insurance plans provide a comprehensive package of benefits, which is set by law. Covered benefits include physician and hospital
services, long-term care, dental care, and prescription drugs. Although extensive prenatal care is credited with Japan's low infant mortality rate, it is
interesting to note that normal childbirth and delivery expenses are not a
covered benefit under the social insurance health plans, because preg-
nancy is not considered a disease. Rather, women typically receive a lump-
sum cash payment that is generally sufficient to cover the cost of medical
services associated with childbirth, while prenatal care is covered by public funds (Jordan 1997; Marmor 1992; Masayana and Campbell 1996;
Yoshikawa and Utsunomiya 1993).

The role of private insurance is limited given that individuals cannot
opt out of the national program, the coverage provided under the plans is
comprehensive, and there is a ceiling on out-of-pocket payments. Private
insurance typically covers supplemental benefits such as private hospital
rooms (though only 10 percent of all hospital rooms are private) and other
amenities during a patient's stay in the hospital (Ikegami 1996).

Health insurance for all those under age 70 is provided through two
major programs, which are both financed through employer–employee
premiums tied to income rather than health status: Employees' Health
Insurance (EHI) covers approximately two-thirds of the population, and
the remaining one-third is covered under the National Health Insurance

(NHI)[3] program. Medical care for all those aged 70 or older (65 if bedridden) is covered by the Roken, a separate system administered by the local governments and financed through a special pooling fund to which all health insurance plans must contribute.

The EHI system provides health insurance coverage to workers and their dependents through health plans managed either by large corporations, known as societies, by the government, or by mutual aid associations. For its part, NHI covers all those not covered by an EHI program, namely the self-employed, owners and employees of firms with fewer than five employees, the unemployed, and retirees. Together, these programs provide health insurance coverage for the entire Japanese population (Table 5–2).[4]

EMPLOYEE HEALTH INSURANCE

Like Germany, Japan has hundreds of insurers. Yet unlike the Germans, the Japanese are not free to choose among insurance funds; rather the choice is made for them depending on the size of the company in which they are employed. Three features distinguish the two major plans for employees and their dependents. First, the government manages the insurance plans for small and medium-sized businesses (with at least 5 and fewer than 700 employees), and larger businesses set up their own separate health insurance plans for their employees. Second, insurance premiums for government-managed insurance are a fixed rate set by law and are shared equally between employer and employee, whereas insurance societies have much broader latitude to set not only the contribution rate but to determine the employer's share of the premium, as described subsequently. Third, government-managed insurance covers only those benefits specified by law, whereas health insurance societies tend to provide additional benefits, such as reimbursement of patient copayments, payment for annual physicals, which are not covered by health insurance, and supplemental cash benefits in the event of illness.

Individuals are not necessarily members of the same insurance plan for life. For instance, a worker may begin her career with a large company and receive insurance coverage through a society-managed health plan. If toward the end of her career she moves to a smaller company, as many Japanese do, she would then be covered under a government-managed insurance plan. At retirement she would receive her health insurance coverage through the NHI program (Yoshikawa and Utsunomiya 1993).

---

[3] Ikegami argues that this translation is misleading and that "Citizens Health Insurance" is a more accurate translation of the program's name.

[4] Fewer than 1 percent of the Japanese population is on public assistance for health care services; this group is not included within this description of the Japanese health care system, nor does it appear in Table 5–2.

TABLE 5–2 Universal health coverage in Japan

Employee health insurance (EHI)	Who is covered	Percentage of the population	Financing	Copayments
Society-managed plans	Workers in large firms (700 or more employees) and their dependents;	26% Enrollees tend to be relatively young and well-paid	Premiums vary by fund, currently averaging 8.39% of salary; employer must pay at least half, but some pay as much as 80%. The government pays all administrative costs.	Employees pay 20% of the cost of inpatient and outpatient services; employee dependents pay 20% of inpatient and 30% of outpatient costs. Out-of pocket costs are capped at approximately $450 per month.
Government-managed plans	Workers in firms with 5 to 300 employees and their dependents are in one national insurance pool.	29% Enrollees tend to be older and less well-paid than those in society-managed plans	Average contribution is fixed by law, currently at 8.5% of wages; split evenly between employer and employee. The government subsidizes 13% of total plan costs	Same
Other: Mutual aid associations (MAA); Seamen's Insurance; Day Laborers' Insurance	MAAs cover national and local public sector employees and their dependents; other plans cover seamen and day workers	MAAs cover 9.5% of the population; other plans 0.5%	8.5% of wages; other plans base premiums on wage level	Same

(Table continues on next page)

TABLE 5-2 (Continued)

Employee health insurance (EHI)	Who is covered	Percentage of the population	Financing	Copayments
National Health (or Citizens' Health) Insurance	All those not covered by EHI: owners of and workers in small firms; the self-employed; the unemployed and retirees and dependents	35% (NHI associations cover the self-employed such as physicians, dentists, hair stylists, etc.) Overall, NHI enrollees tend to be older, lower income people.	Premiums based on income and assets take the form of a NHI tax; annual household premiums averaged $1,140 in 1996. National tax revenues cover 50%.	Employees and dependents pay 30% of all in-patient and outpatient costs; retirees pay 20%.
Health Services for the Elderly (Roken)	Persons aged 70 and older (or 65 and older if bedridden)		Nearly two-thirds of the financing comes from employment-based insurance plans and nearly one-third from national and local government funds, with 4% coming from patient co-payments.	Patients pay 500 yen per physician visit and 1,000 yen per day for hospital care.

The groups covered under the EHI and NHI programs are described next, as are the financing arrangements for each insurance program.

SOCIETY-MANAGED HEALTH PLANS. Larger companies set up their own independent health insurance plans for their employees, known as *kempo kumiais,* or health insurance societies. These societies can be either single-employer plans or multiemployer plans when the combined number of employees is 700 or more. The societies, which numbered 1,815 as of 1995, are managed by representatives of labor and management. They provide coverage to more than one quarter of the population. These societies go beyond merely covering the costs of health care, however, as noted by Wolfson and Levin:

> One of the mottos of Japanese companies . . . "the company is people"— recognizes the value of each employee as a company asset. A healthy, well-informed employee is seen as the most important investment a company can have. The kempos are the principal social and economic vehicles for helping to make this happen. (1986, 39)

Though private, the societies are unlike private insurance groups in the United States, as they are only allowed to function as an alternative to the government-managed plan and are subject to governmental oversight and regulation through the Ministry of Health and Welfare (Horkitz 1990). As separate legal entities, the societies' assets are kept apart from the corporation's and cannot be used for anything other than to pay health care bills. The fact that the list of covered services is set by law limits employers' ability to tinker with the contents of the benefits packages offered to employees (Ikegami 1991).

Health insurance premiums are income based and paid by employers and employees. The employer share, which varies by fund, must be at least 50 percent of total premium contributions, but can be as high as 80 percent in some companies. The employee share is in the form of a payroll tax deducted from a worker's paycheck as part of the overall Social Security payment (Ikegami 1991). Premium contribution rates vary among health insurance societies, ranging from less than 7 to more than 9.5 percent of wages (Figure 5–3). As of the fall of 1997, the average contribution rate was 8.39 percent of wages.

Health insurance premium rates in firms with older workforces, such as those in the steel industry, as well as those with lower wage workers, such as in the textile industry, tend to be higher relative to other firms (Ikegami 1991, 1996). For instance, at NEC Corporation where the average employee age was 30.4 years, health insurance premiums were 7.0 percent of wages, with 4.2 percent covered by the employer and 2.8 percent by the employee. Kawasaki Steel's average employee age, in contrast, was 43.1 years and the premium contribution rate was 8.8 percent, with the

FIGURE 5-3   Contribution Rates under Japanese Society-Managed Health Insurance
(contribution rate as percentage of pay)

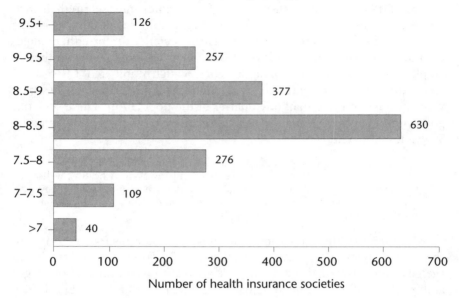

Number of health insurance societies

Source: Social Insurance Agency, Outline of Social Insurance in Japan, 1996.

employer paying 5.6 and the employee 3.2 percent of wages (Yoshikawa
and Utsonomiya 1993).[5]

In addition to premiums, employees are also subject to copayments.
Health care reforms implemented in the fall of 1997 doubled the amount
of out-of-pocket costs employees were to shoulder, from 10 to 20 percent
of inpatient and outpatient costs. Employees' dependents pay 20 percent
of the cost of inpatient care and 30 percent of outpatient care. The copayments for all EHI plans are limited by a ceiling on out-of-pocket payments
of 63,600 yen per month (approximately $450).[6] All costs beyond that
ceiling are reimbursed by the plans.

GOVERNMENT-MANAGED HEALTH PLANS. Employees of small and
medium-sized businesses (between 5 and 300 employees) receive coverage through a nationwide government-managed health insurance plan run
by the central government's Social Insurance Agency (SIA)—the largest insurer in Japan. These government-managed plans operate out of the SIA's
network of nearly 300 local offices.

---

[5] Data for 1990.

[6] All dollar values in this chapter are based on June 1, 1998, exchange rate of 139.57 yen to the
dollar.

Contributions to government-managed health insurance, like society-managed insurance, are income based, but the contribution rate is fixed by the Ministry of Health and Welfare within the range of 6.6 to 9.1 percent of pay. The 1997 reforms raised the contribution rate from 8.2 to 8.5 percent of pay, split equally between employer and employee. The same copayment rates and ceilings on out-of-pocket payments for society-managed insurance pertain to government-managed insurance.

In an effort to equalize the cost burden across the various plans, the central government provides a subsidy to the government-managed plans since their members, as employees of small and medium-sized companies, tend to be less well-off than those working for larger companies covered by society-managed plans. As of 1996 the government subsidy covered 13 percent of the government-managed insurance plan's overall expenditures (Social Insurance Agency 1996).

MUTUAL AID ASSOCIATIONS AND OTHER INSURANCE GROUPS. Mutual aid associations provide coverage for public employees, both national and local, including public and private school teachers and staff. The average premium contribution rate is 8.5 percent of wages.

A small specialized group of people who work on crews of ships are covered by Seamen's Insurance, and workers hired by the day and expected to work for fewer than two months, such as construction workers, for instance, are covered by Day Laborer's Insurance; premiums vary according to wage level.

NATIONAL HEALTH INSURANCE

The one-third of the population that is not covered by employment-based plans receives coverage through the National Health Insurance program. The NHI program, administered by the municipal governments and NHI associations, provides coverage to the unemployed, owners and employees of businesses with fewer than five employees, retirees previously covered under employee insurance, the self-employed, and the dependents of all these individuals. The self-employed tend to be covered by NHI associations that insure individuals in the same occupation such as farmers, barbers, carpenters, as well as physicians, dentists, and lawyers (Ikegami 1991; Powell and Anesaki 1990).[7]

NHI premiums are calculated on the basis of household income and assets and take the form of a local NHI tax. In 1996 the ceiling on annual premiums was 530,000 yen per household (approximately $3,800) and the average annual household premium was 158,580 yen (approximately $1,140; Social Insurance Agency 1996). Employees and their dependents

---

[7] As of March 1995 there were 166 of these NHI associations.

pay 30 percent of all inpatient and outpatient costs, and retirees pay 20 percent of these costs. Though the copayments are higher than under employee health insurance, the same monthly ceiling on out-of-pocket payments pertains. The national government provides a subsidy to the NHI that covers one-half of the plan's total expenditures—in essence, the government pays the employer's share of the premium for NHI enrollees (J. Campbell 1996).

HEALTH CARE FOR THE ELDERLY

These descriptions have provided a picture of health insurance provision to all individuals under the age of 70. A law enacted in 1972 entitled all Japanese citizens over the age of 70 (age 65 if bedridden) to free medical care through the health insurance system. The cost of this free care was to be shared by the different insurance schemes, but because of demographic factors, the NHI program had a disproportionate share of elderly members and therefore carried most of the financial burden. This burden became impossible to maintain as NHI's share of costs for the elderly increased from 20.8 percent in 1973 to more than 32 percent in 1981 (Steslicke 1989).

These financial pressures culminated in the 1982 Health Care for the Elderly law. This law determined that the health care costs of the most expensive portion of the population would be paid for not by raising the copayment and premium rates of the elderly (which were and still are marginal). Rather, the government created a system of transfer payments from employee health insurance plans, essentially shifting resources from the healthy and wealthy, and thereby spreading the cost burden across a broader section of the population.

The vehicle for this transfer payment system was a separate insurance pooling fund to which each insurance plan must contribute a set amount. That the society-managed health plans were generating large budget surpluses at that time played no small role in the selection of this funding approach. The contribution amount, rather than being a reflection of the share of elderly members in a particular fund, is calculated based on the ratio of elderly persons in the entire population. In this way, no single fund bears a larger share of the cost than any other fund (J. Campbell 1996).

The mandatory contributions from the health insurance plans cover approximately two-thirds of the cost of care for elderly individuals, and the national and local governments provide 20 and 10 percent of the financing, respectively. Finally, small copayments on the part of elderly people fill in the remaining 4 to 5 percent of expenditures. The current cost-sharing requirement is less than $10 per month for outpatient care (regardless of the number of visits) and $6 per day for hospital care. This in a land where a typical cup of coffee costs $3.50.

Reforms implemented in 1997 have changed the copayment structure; instead of paying a fixed-sum payment per month, patients will pay 500 yen per outpatient visit. Hospital charges were increased from the current rate of 710 yen per day to 1,000 yen with an additional increase to 1,200 yen in 1999 (Spencer and Associates 1997).

Although the society-managed plans were running surpluses in the early 1980s and could therefore afford to spread the wealth, so to speak, more than two-thirds of the health insurance societies of the fifty largest employers had a deficit in fiscal year 1996. The societies attributed their financial woes to the hefty contribution to the health care program for elderly individuals, and nearly three quarters of all societies responding to a national survey supported halting that contribution. Government-managed plans, for their part, are not in any better financial condition; they have been running a deficit since 1993 (Spencer and Associates 1997).

HEALTH CARE DELIVERY

The Japanese health care delivery system is predominantly private, with 81 percent of all hospitals and 94 percent of all physician offices under private ownership (Ikegami 1996).

HOSPITALS AND CLINICS

The most distinguishing feature of the Japanese delivery system is the absence of a clear functional separation between hospital and clinics. Clinics are essentially extensions of a physician's solo practice and are distinguishable from hospitals in many cases only by the legal definition that states that clinics are facilities with fewer than twenty inpatient beds, whereas hospitals have more than twenty beds. A large share of the hospitals are small physician-owned facilities that have outgrown the twenty-bed limit. Indeed, up until the mid-1980s clinics could freely add beds until they became small hospitals; the result of this laissez-faire approach to hospital capacity is that with 16 beds per 1,000 population, Japan has more hospital beds per capita than any other industrialized nation. Such unbridled expansion was halted by a 1985 amendment to the Medical Services Act that require local governments to prepare regional health care plans to control hospital capacity. It is now extremely difficult to build new hospitals in urban areas in Japan (Yoshikawa 1993).

The majority of hospitals are privately owned; slightly more than 80 percent of all hospitals and 70 percent of all hospital beds are under private ownership, with the largest share of hospitals owned by private insurance associations (Figure 5–4). These private hospitals are known as

FIGURE 5-4   Hospitals by Ownership, Japan 1990 (as percentage)

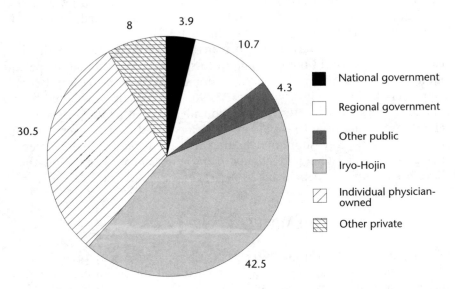

Source: Yoshikawa, Bhattacharva, and Vost (eds.) *Health Economics of Japan.* Tokyo: University of Tokyo Press, 1996.

iryo-hojin hospitals after the special legal status accorded such nonprofit facilities in the health care sector. Japanese law prohibits investor-owned, for-profit hospitals. Though the law bars private hospitals from distributing profits to outside shareholders, it does allow profits to be earned for the purpose of reinvestment. Profits may be used, for example, to expand a hospital's services. Thus these private hospitals are nonprofit institutions to the extent that they are not financially accountable to stockholders, yet physicians who own and operate their own hospitals are clearly interested in their financial sustainability (Abe 1985; Iglehart 1988b; Murdo 1989; Powell and Anesaki 1990; Yoshikawa, Bhattacharya, and Vogt 1996). The regulation forbidding the distribution of dividends and profits to outside shareholders has limited the development of multihospital systems in Japan (Ikegami 1996).

Clinics and hospitals compete for patients, and the competition is heightened by the fact that clinic physicians do not have hospital-admitting privileges, so they cannot follow their patients when they are admitted to the hospital for care. Hospitals employ their own physicians on fixed salaries and run large ambulatory care facilities (Ikegami 1991). Because clinics compete with hospitals for patients, there tends to be much duplication of equipment, as both facilities invest in the latest medical technology to attract patients. Moreover, the lack of a formal separation between hospitals and clinics results in redundant testing as procedures are started anew as a patient who had been treated in a clinic enters the hospital.

The public-sector university hospitals have only one-third of all hospital beds, yet perform nearly three quarters of all the operations requiring general anesthesia.[8] This is in large part a result of the fact that the most advanced medical equipment is centralized in the larger public hospitals because they receive government subsidies for capital improvements that the small private hospitals do not (Ikegami and Campbell 1995).

The hospital picture is further muddled by the fact that there is no true functional difference between acute care hospitals and long-term care hospitals. Given the small number of long-term care facilities, many hospitals have become de facto nursing homes. More than 40 percent of hospital inpatients are over the age of 65, and, at any one time, nearly half of them have been in the hospital for more than six months (Ikegami and Campbell 1995). Though a new category of specialized hospitals dealing with chronic diseases has been developed, many general hospitals still provide long-term care services.[9]

Another distinguishing characteristic of the Japanese hospital sector is that Japanese law requires that all chief executive officers (medical directors) of all hospitals and clinics be physicians. These physician-executives have administrative as well as medical responsibilities, but many lack the necessary background and formal training in hospital administration and management (Iglehart 1988b; Ikegami 1991; Levin, Wolfson, and Akiyama 1987; Murdo 1989; Powell and Anesaki 1990).

PHYSICIANS

Physicians in Japan are divided into two groups: Approximately one-third are private practitioners paid on a fee-for-service basis, and the remainder are hospital-based physicians on salary. Regardless of the type of health insurance plan, patients have unrestricted access to virtually all physicians without an initial referral.

The composition of the physician population is changing as the traditional clinic doctor is gradually being replaced by younger, hospital-based doctors. Whereas 45 percent of all doctors owned clinics in 1960, fewer than 30 percent did in 1990. Hospital doctors have assumed an in-

---

[8] Public hospitals tend to be larger, with an average of 286 beds versus an average of 141 beds in private hospitals (Yoshikawa, Bhattacharya, and Vogt 1996).
[9] I am grateful to Mr. Kazuhito Ihara, director of the Health and Welfare Department, JETRO, for pointing this out to me.

creasing share of the physician population, growing from 44 percent of all physicians in 1960 to 67 percent in 1990 (Yoshikawa et al. 1996).

Unlike in the United States, primary care physicians in private practice earn approximately twice that of specialists employed by hospitals. Hospital doctors' lower incomes are counterbalanced by the fact that they are held in higher esteem by society than private practitioners (Ikegami 1991; Ikegami and Campbell 1995; Marmor 1992).

CONTROLLING HEALTH CARE COSTS: NATIONWIDE FEE SCHEDULE

Whereas one has to look hard to find much regulation on the delivery side of Japanese health care, regulation looms large on the financing side. A nationwide fee schedule determines payment for all outpatient and inpatient medical services. All Japanese health care providers are reimbursed according to a procedure-based fee schedule (similar to Medicare's resource-based relative value scale), known as the point-fee system. More than 3,000 medical procedures, services, and products are listed and given a specific number of points, with one point equal to 10 yen.[10] A separate drug tariff lists the prices of more than 13,000 drugs. The point-fee system reimburses hospitals according to a standard per diem rate.

Everyone pays the same fee for the same service, regardless of whether it was performed in an urban hospital or rural clinic and regardless of what type of physician performed it. Essentially, the flow of all health care payments to multiple insurers are controlled by one spigot—the national fee schedule. Moreover, physicians must accept the fee as payment in full; billing beyond the fixed price is not allowed. Benefits are set by law and all payers receive the same payment for the same service (Iglehart 1988b; Ikegami 1991, 1996; Ikegami and Campbell 1995; Powell and Anesaki 1990; White 1995).

Utilization review exists, but the Japanese version entails health care bills being submitted monthly to a regional office of a central fund for employer-based plans and a central fund for National Health Insurance. A panel of physicians reviews bills to check for overutilization. Given the sheer volume of the claims, however, each reviewer spends an average of 10 seconds on each individual bill. On approval at the central fund level, bills are sent to the individual health plans for payment (Okimato and Yoshikawa 1993; White 1995).

The fee schedule is revised every two years based on recommendations of *Chuikyo*, an advisory body to the Ministry of Health and Welfare

---

[10] In 1990, for example, an initial physician consultation was worth 30 points, an MRI scan 2,100 points, and an appendectomy 4,800 points (Yoshikawa et al. 1996).

known as the Central Social Insurance Medical Council. The twenty-member council includes eight representatives of health care providers (five physicians, two dentists, and one pharmacist, but is notably lacking in any direct representatives of the hospital sector),[11] eight payers (four insurers, two management, and two labor), and four consumers (one lawyer and three economists to represent the public interest; Ikegami and Campbell 1995), and bears a distinct resemblance to Germany's Concerted Action.

The powerful Japan Medical Association dominates the provider side and nominates the provider representatives, and in so doing has managed to keep any representatives of the Japan Hospital Association off the council (Ikegami 1991). It is therefore not surprising that the fee schedule favors physicians in private practice over hospital physicians—in other words, fees are low for surgery and intensive care. Such lower fees combined with a strong cultural aversion to invasive procedures may be the reason that surgery rates in Japan are significantly lower than those in the United States (Ikegami and Campbell 1995; White 1995).

Japan's health care budget is set through a two-step process. First, a cap on the overall annual increase in health care expenditure—what essentially amounts to a global budget—is determined in negotiations between the Ministry of Finance and the Ministry of Health and Welfare. The Ministry of Finance is involved because government subsidies to the health insurance plans are a fixed share of the plans' overall expenditures, so if the plans' cost increases, so does the government subsidy. After these negotiations to basically determine the size of the overall health care pie are complete, the Ministry of Health and Welfare, based on the Council's recommendations, determines how that pie should be divided—in other words, the specific details of the fee schedule (Ikegami 1996; Masayuma and Campbell 1996).

When the fee schedule is revised, changes are not made across the board by simply changing the factor used to convert points to yen; rather, the fee schedule is adjusted procedure by procedure. But such adjustments are not made lightly: Any increase in the price of a covered service, or the addition of a service or procedure, yields a large cost increase because all services are available to the entire population not just to a small select group or to those who can afford any additional service. And because the government's expenditures increase when total expenditures increase, the government has a strong incentive to keep a lid on costs (J. Campbell 1996; Ikegami 1996; Ikegami and Campbell 1995).

---

[11] Thus the large public teaching hospitals that perform most specialty medicine and surgery are not represented on the council.

THE SUN ALSO SETS ON JAPANESE HEALTH CARE

Japanese health care expenditures have remained relatively constant as a percentage of GDP, hovering around the 7 percent mark throughout the 1980s and into the 1990s. Such stability in health care expenditures has been maintained by a well-oiled economic machine that hummed along at high rates of growth, fueling rising incomes. But current conditions are troubling to say the least. Japan's economy is now experiencing a negative growth rate for the first time in twenty-five years. Demographically Japan is a very old nation, with the number of people aged 65 or older surpassing those under age 15; birth rates are below the level needed to replace the population. Needless to say, these factors have led to increased financial pressures on the Japanese health care system, and will continue to do so in the future.

Health care spending in Japan increased 6 percent between fiscal years 1995 and 1996. The Ministry of Health and Welfare attributed this increase to costs for health care for elderly individuals, which rose nearly 10 percent from 1995 to 1996 (Marketletter 1997b). Health care expenditures for elderly individuals already make up nearly 37 percent of total health spending, and the share of the population age 65 and older has not even reached the 17 percent mark, not to mention the 25 percent level it will hit in 2020.

Increasing cost pressures are evident in the fact that more than 70 percent of all health insurance societies suffered losses in 1996 and have been forced to raise their premium rates. The government-managed insurance program also faces financial pressures and suffered the largest deficit in history in fiscal year 1996. Given that health care expenditures are financed to a large extent out of payroll taxes, slow wage growth has a particularly deleterious effect on health care financing, necessitating premium increases and higher patient copayments for services and prescription drugs.

The ability of the Japanese health care system to respond to the challenges of an aging population and rising health care costs will be constrained by certain cultural characteristics. Japan is referred to as "a dynamic society without change" (Hashimoto 1984, 335)—or, in the words of a more contemporary critic, "Today's aging Japanese, formed by an antiquated, inward-looking, ultimately self-defeating system, have no idea how to change it—or whether they even want to" (Sayle 1998). Entrenched resistance to change will make it difficult to address many of the health care system's underlying weaknesses.

AREAS FOR REFORM

Some of the more significant problems facing Japan's health care system include quality of care, overprescription of drugs, lack of functional differentiation between clinics and hospitals, and excessively long average length of hospital stay primarily as a result of the shortage of long-term care facilities.

QUALITY OF CARE. Quality-related problems within the Japanese health care system include the conditions of Japanese hospitals, which would be considered spartan by U.S. standards. Facilities are short on amenities, privacy, and space, with patients generally placed in wards of six to eight people (Rodwin 1994). In addition, long waiting times to see a doctor are common because patients are seen on a first-come, first-served basis. The term *3-for-3 shuffle* is used to describe a patient waiting three hours for three minutes with the doctor (R. Campbell 1996). Long waiting times are particularly acute in the large public and teaching hospitals that are perceived to offer higher quality care (Calhoun 1993; Ikegami 1996). In some cases patients offer financial gifts or "tips" to physicians to get special attention or quicker service (Ikegami and Campbell 1995), but typically these gifts or tips are offered to the physician after the course of treatment and are a generally accepted practice of supplementing physician fees.

Another quality issue is the paucity of information shared with patients. Japanese doctors do not disclose much information about a patient's condition, nor do they explain medical procedures. Patients rarely question the physician, reflecting entrenched deference to the "revered status of the Sensei" (teacher or master; Calhoun 1993, 260). And the Japanese courts support this absence of informed consent, having ruled on a case in the early 1990s that a physician was not required to give a cancer patient the full details of his condition (Calhoun 1993; Rodwin 1994).[12]

There is no formal system of quality control and monitoring nor of board certification, and the powerful Japan Medical Association has successfully championed and guarded physician autonomy, staving off any form of third-party intervention. No significant peer review exists as physicians in Japan do not welcome other professionals monitoring their activities (Calhoun 1993; Rodwin 1994).

Many observers trace quality problems to the fee-schedule-based reimbursement method. Because all providers are paid the same fee for the same service, regardless of quality, no incentives exist to guarantee or improve the quality of care. Indeed, there is no direct relationship between a physician's training and salary level. As noted earlier, salaried hospital physicians (who are often better trained) earn significantly less than private practitioners (Ikegami 1991; Marmor 1992; Powell and Anesaki 1990).

As a consequence of binding limits on physicians' fees and low reimbursement rates for office visits, many physicians "game the system" by

---

[12] The government's Medical Care Insurance System Reform Council's August 1997 report, National Health Care for the 21st Century, specifically lists informed consent as an area that will receive increased attention.

increasing the volume of services. Clinic doctors see from 49 to 100 out-patients per day for an average of three to five minutes; doctors visits tend to focus more on curative treatments such as prescription drugs than preventive care (Ikegami 1991; Powell and Anesaki 1990). Because consultations times are short, patients go the doctor more frequently. In 1995, for example, annual physician consultations in Japan approached sixteen visits per person, compared to approximately six in the United States, Germany, and the United Kingdom (OECD 1998).

Such high rates of physician contact may be driven down as the greater cost burden is increasingly felt by patients. For example, according to a survey by the *Nikkei Weekly*, not long after the September 1997 reforms doubled the patients' copayment rate to 20 percent of costs, medical institutions noted a decline in outpatient visits (*Nikkei Weekly* 1997).

Physicians also compensate for low fees by prescribing more medicines or ordering more tests that carry a higher point value (Abe 1985; Ikegami 1991; Murdo 1989). Moreover, the "dual role of the individual practitioner—doctor and businessman—gives rise to some dubious medical practices and conflicts of interest" (Powell and Anesaki 1990, 234).

PHYSICIANS AS PHARMACISTS. Nowhere is this conflict of interest more apparent than in the fact that physicians simultaneously prescribe and dispense prescription drugs. Thus we can add physician–pharmacist to the physician–businessperson role in the Japanese system. A significant portion of a physician's income is derived from dispensing drugs, which is one of the primary reasons Japan leads the world in per capita prescription drug consumption. Pharmaceuticals represented fully one-fifth of total health expenditures in Japan in 1994, compared to 8 percent in the United States (OECD 1998).

The Ministry of Health and Welfare sets official drug prices through the government price schedule. Doctors, however, negotiate with drug companies and purchase prescription drugs at discounted rates. Doctors are reimbursed the full official price, however, and keep the difference—known as *Yakkasa* or the "doctor's margin"—between the discounted price and the official reimbursement price. But physicians view the substantial margin, which amounts to approximately 26 percent and has been estimated to run as high as $9 billion a year (*Marketletter* 1997a) as fair compensation for low fees for their services.

The profit incentive in prescribing leads physicians to prescribe large amounts of expensive drugs, because the higher the price, the bigger the margin. Moreover, physicians are required by law to dispense limited amounts of pharmaceuticals, so each time the patient returns to refill his or her prescription, the doctor pockets an additional dispensing fee (Eisenstodt 1992; Powell and Anesaki 1990; White 1995). Dutch journalist Karel van Wolferen, writing in his influential and controversial book, *The*

Enigma of Japanese Power, noted that this practice has led to "corrupt relations with the pharmaceutical industry, to an alarming degree of overmedication, and to some very rich doctors" (1989, 54). Indeed, the practice of overprescription of drugs is so widespread in Japan that it has given rise to its own phrase: *kusuri zuke,* literally translated as "pickling with drugs" (Powell and Anesaki 1990, 174). This is not only a financing problem but a medical one as well, because overprescribing limits the ability of drugs to fight certain strains of bacteria (Ikegami and Campbell 1995).

The government has responded to this situation by significantly reducing the fee schedule prices for drugs. Between 1981 and 1992, the average price of drugs fell by more than half, bringing down pharmaceutical's share in overall health care expenditures from a whopping 44 percent in 1980 to 20 percent in 1992 (Ikegami and Campbell 1995). The government has continued to pare down the official reimbursement prices of drugs covered by health insurance, reducing prices by an average of 8.5 percent in 1996, followed by another price reduction of an average of 4.4 percent in 1997 (*Med Ad News* 1997).

Reforms proposed in the fall of 1997 called for replacing the official government-mandated drug-pricing system with a reference price system by 2000. The government would classify drugs in groups according to their effective ingredients and would set a standard reference drug price. Patients would be required to pay any additional cost beyond the reference price (Spencer and Associates 1997). The reference price would act as a ceiling, effectively crowding out the doctor's margin.

Reforms implemented in 1997 introduced additional copayments for patients taking more than one type of prescription drug, ranging from 30 yen if a patient is taking two to three prescription drugs per day to 100 yen for six or more drugs. It is hoped that the combination of increased copayment rates and the proposed reference prices will raise patients' awareness of prescription drug prices and discourage overprescription by physicians. Moreover, the government is planning to take steps to separate drug prescription from dispensing and to improve the quality of pharmacists so that they may take over the dispensing role (Government of Japan 1997).

COMPETING HOSPITALS AND CLINICS. Excess capacity in the hospital sector is a serious problem: There are too many hospitals, too many beds, and the per diem reimbursement rate encourages clinics and hospitals to keep the beds filled. Moreover, because the majority of Japanese hospitals and clinics are privately run and many are physician-owned, physicians clearly have little interest in referring patients to their competitors or allowing physicians who are not salaried employees of the hospital to have admitting privileges in their hospitals. Keeping the system closed precludes any organized system of patient referral and ensures much duplication of tests, procedures, and equipment.[13] This is particularly the case as physicians own much of the medical equipment in Japan, so there is a powerful financial incentive to order more tests and procedures. Indeed, in the absence of any limits on acquisition of technology there has been a proliferation of highly advanced medical equipment in Japan. Consider the case of computerized tomography (CT) scanners. In 1982 Japan had 18.5 CT scanners per million people, compared to 10.7 in the United States, 2.1 in West Germany, 3.1 in Canada, and 5.7 in the Netherlands. Whereas there was a total of 664 whole-body CT scanners in Japan in 1981, this number increased five-fold by 1987 (Abe 1985; Marmor 1992; Murdo 1991; Powell and Anesaki 1990).

A 1992 amendment to the Medical Services Act represented an attempt to formally delineate the roles of clinics and hospitals. Revisions in the fee schedule were introduced to use financial incentives to clarify hospitals' roles as providers of inpatient care and clinics as providers of outpatient care.

PROLONGED HOSPITAL STAYS. Hospitals in Japan differ from those in the United States and other Western nations in that chronically ill patients who would normally be put in nursing homes in other countries are treated as inpatients in Japanese hospitals. This practice of keeping geriatric, long-term patients in hospitals, known as social hospitalization, is reflected in average length of hospital stay, which is more than five times longer than the average hospital stay in the United States and considerably longer than that of other nations.

Social hospitalization is the result of the slow development of nursing homes in Japan, which stems from cultural factors including a strong sense of responsibility to one's family (Hashimoto 1984). A social stigma is attached to institutionalization, which is often compared with the ancient practice of *ubasuteyama,* or leaving one's family member on the mountain to die (EBRI 1989; Murdo 1989).

Japanese traditional norms place the responsibility of caring for elderly parents on the daughter-in-law. Yet with increased longevity, many of the daughters-in-law are themselves elderly and in need of care. At the same time, an increasing share of younger women are joining the paid labor force[14] (Ihara 1997; Ikegami 1997; Matsunuga 1997). Finally, many young women are choosing not to marry—currently two-thirds of all Japanese women between the ages of 20 and 30 have never married (Sayle

---

[13] Ikegami has pointed out that an effective referral system requires procedures to evaluate the quality of care and that this would in turn require "information disclosure and a formal system of external audit, concepts that are foreign to Japanese culture, and especially so in health care" (Ikegami 1996, 17).

[14] The labor force participation rate of women rose from 57 percent in 1984 to 62 percent in 1994.

1998). Finally, societal attitudes are changing toward the "feudalistic belief" that the daughter-in-law be the defacto caretaker of aging parents
(Ihara 1998, 6).

The government launched a ten-year strategy in 1989 known as the
"Gold Plan," aimed at improving and expanding health care services for
elderly individuals. The plan set goals to increase home care services,
nursing home beds, and other forms of housing for the elderly. Increased
funding was made available in the 1994 new Gold Plan; in all more than
$70 billion will be invested over the 1989–1999 period. The number of
nursing homes has grown under the Gold Plan, but still falls far short of
demand; in the urban areas, the waiting time for admission to a nursing
home can be as long as several years (Ikegami 1997).

In addition to the Gold Plan, the government passed a new long-term
care insurance program in 1997 to take effect in 2000. Japan thus joins the
Netherlands and Germany in establishing public long-term care insurance
programs. Japan's long-term care program will cover institutional care in
geriatric hospitals and other hospitals designed for elderly patients, nursing homes and group homes, as well as home-help services, day care, and
loan of medical devices (i.e., wheelchairs). Though the payment for institutional care will include the fees for physicians' services, any ambulatory
care rendered in physicians' offices and hospitals will continue to be covered by the existing health insurance system.

The new long-term care insurance program will be financed half by
premium contributions and the other half by general tax revenues. Each
individual aged 40 and older will make a mandatory premium contribution; as with health insurance, premiums will take the form of payroll deductions, with the employer paying half of the premium. Retirees' contributions will be deducted from their pension payments, and those with low
incomes will pay reduced rates. The monthly payment initially will be
2,500 yen (approximately $20). Patients will also pay a 10 percent copay-
ment at the time of service.

The remaining half of the program's finances will come from the three
levels of government: the national government will pay 50 percent and the
prefectures and municipalities will pay 25 percent each. To make sure that
no one municipality carries a heavier financial burden, the premium contributions from individuals aged 40 to 64 will all go into a national pool
and then be distributed to each municipality. The municipalities (cities,
towns, and villages), which already act as health insurers for retirees, will
administer the long-term care program (Ikegami 1997).

Private firms are already jockeying for position in the new long-term
care marketplace, competing on the basis of price. The company Life
Commune, for example, slashed the required up-front residency fee in its
three recently opened nursing homes from an industry average of 27 mil-

lion yen to 5 million yen (approximately $38,500; Nihon Kezai Shimbun, cited in AARP 1998).

THE ENIGMA OF JAPANESE HEALTH CARE

The Japanese health care system is indeed a puzzle with many confusing pieces. The health care system is largely private in financing and delivery yet features a heavy dose of governmental regulations—the government not only sets the price of most health care services and products, it regulates the insurers and determines what is to be covered. The system provides universal coverage and health care services that have at least indirectly led to good health outcomes and has done so at a relatively low cost. Yet there are significant quality problems and other weaknesses and distortions in the system that set off alarm bells. As one analyst has suggested, Americans should perhaps "take advantage of their position as 'health insurance laggards' to study and reflect critically on the experience of Japan" (Steslicke 1982, 197).

Japan, like Germany, gradually phased in insurance coverage, which is now provided to the entire population. And in Japan, as in Germany and Canada, universal coverage and a private delivery system coexist with strict governmental regulation and cost-control mechanisms.

As noted at the outset of this chapter, any attempts to apply lessons drawn from the Japanese health care experience to the U.S. health care system must first take into account vast differences in the composition of Japanese and American societies as well as other cultural and economic factors. Simply put, the stresses, demands, and pressures on the U.S. system are not directly comparable with those on the Japanese system (Ikegami 1991). And if the reaction to the Clinton health care plan is any indication, the heavy hand of government in the Japanese health care system would not likely receive a warm U.S. welcome. Yet despite these differences—and the serious challenges facing the Japanese system, it is possible to glean several potential lessons from the Japanese experience.

By virtue of its rapidly aging population, Japan has a leg up on the United States in the area of health-related policies for the aging. The United States and Japan are facing the same pressures of how to distribute the financial burden of health care for a growing elderly population. We have seen that Japan has responded to the challenge of its aging population through the ten-year Gold Plan, followed by the new long-term care insurance program slated to take effect in 2000. Moreover, Japan's experience with pooling risk is significant: The government uses general revenues to provide subsidies to funds with a higher ratio of low-income or high-risk members, which tend to be elderly individuals (White 1995). In addition, recent reforms have required elderly people to shoulder a larger share of their health care costs.

The egalitarian nature of Japanese health care—itself a direct reflection of Japanese culture—is achieved through direct subsidies of the old by the young, combined with income-based premiums and government subsidies to lower-income groups. Everyone receives essentially the same benefits, and no one is allowed to opt out of the system. Moreover, the fee schedule, which ensures all providers are paid the same for the same service, combined with mandatory coverage, essentially eliminates any need to cherry-pick among patients according to risk.

The structure of the Japanese health care system has also enabled Japan to benefit from administrative cost savings. The health care claims processing system is simplified by mandatory coverage and uniform fees, which preclude any haggling over what is or is not covered. Moreover, because health care consumers have no real choice of insurance plan, insurers' marketing costs are limited (Ikegami 1991).

This overview of Japanese health care reveals that health care costs in Japan are controlled through governmental oversight of a system in which care is essentially privately financed and delivered. Employers and employees contribute toward the cost of health insurance, and government subsidizes a significant portion of insurance costs. All parties, therefore, have a shared interest in cost containment (Murdo 1989). In Japan, as in Germany, Canada, and other nations, binding fee schedules govern physician reimbursement (as well as hospital fees in Japan). Although physician and hospital payment levels are set by the government, there is significant input from payers and providers through their representation on the Council.

CONVERGENCE

Mitsuru Fujii and Michael Reich have identified several broad patterns in Japanese health policy that are similar to trends within the health care systems of other nations. The first observation is that the 1980s witnessed an increase in government regulation in the health care arena. This trend is clear in Japan, where government regulation and oversight looms large within the health care system.

The government's role can be expected to remain strong, and even get an added boost by the ebbing influence of the Japan Medical Association (JMA). As the number of clinic-based physicians—the JMA's core constituency—continues to lose ground to hospital-based physicians, the power of the JMA will decrease commensurately (Yoshikawa 1992). Moreover, the consensus within the JMA has eroded as various factions are pursuing differing goals (Maurer 1996).

Parallel with this development is the continued, and indeed heightened, emphasis on cost control at work in most industrialized nations, which has taken precedence over such health care goals as improving quality, and in the case of the United States, expanded access. Fujii and Reich also observe that medical services policy has taken a back seat to health insurance policy, which is in turn driven by economic factors. The introduction of increased patient cost-sharing in Japan, for example, is more a response to fiscal realities than a goal of medical services policy. Health insurance policy in Japan, as in many nations, has been essentially reactive in nature; changes in policy occur as a result of socioeconomic developments and political pressures, and are not based on long-range planning toward some desired medical goal (Fujii and Reich 1988).

Thus as the health care systems of different nations experience the same pressures and face similar problems, it is likely that there will be further signs of convergence toward common ground—such as increased governmental regulation over privately based systems that will call increasingly on health care consumers to shoulder more of the burden of health care costs.

Another area of limited convergence between the Japanese and the U.S. systems is the experimentation in Japan with a fixed fee per treatment for certain diseases, somewhat akin to the use of diagnosis-related groups in the U.S. Medicare system. The Ministry of Health is considering a program of fixed fees per treatment of each disease in ten trial hospitals.

Further signs of limited convergence may be the development of a greater role for private insurance in Japan. Increasing patient cost burdens may fuel this demand. Any changes will be clearly limited by the long-held cultural preferences of Japanese society. Ikegami has observed that the Japanese public would find it "morally reprehensible to have a diversity of services based on willingness (or ability to pay)" and that "a blatantly two-tiered system would be difficult to implement in a country of Japan's economic and social homogeneity" (Ikegami 1991, 105).

Managed care in the U.S. fashion has yet to establish a beachhead on the island nation, and noted health economist Naoki Ikegami, like others, wonders whether letting the managed care genie out of the bottle in Japan would be worth the tradeoffs in terms of micromanagement and potential limits on services. Significant obstacles to the development of managed care practices include the absence of standardization of procedures; Japanese physicians are not accustomed to treating patients according to standard protocols or guidelines. Patients for their part are accustomed to free access to physicians and would balk at any attempts to curtail such freedom.[15]

Yet Japan may look to the tools of managed care to address the pressing needs of quality monitoring, assessment, and improvement through disease management and utilization review. Japan may also turn to such managed-care techniques as the use of gatekeepers and referral systems to control access to hospitals and specialists.

---

[15] I am grateful to Mr. Kazuhito Ihara for these points.

CHAPTER 6

Northern Exposure: Canada's National Health Insurance System

Canada's single-payer universal coverage health care system, known as Medicare, played a prominent role as a potential model for reform in the U.S. health care debate in the early 1990s. Though Canada's health care system has since faded from U.S. headlines, it remains an important reminder of the accomplishment of universal health coverage north of the U.S. border.

Canada and the United States, more so than other nations in this study, share similar cultures, economies, geographic characteristics, and, for the most part, languages and decentralized federal–provincial/state systems of government. The U.S. and Canadian health care systems were once quite similar, but since the early 1970s Canada has taken the path of universal health insurance, with the provincial governments the sole payers of publicly financed health care services for all medically necessary services. Canada distinguishes itself from other industrialized nations in that private insurers are not permitted to offer coverage for services provided under the provincial health plans.

More than a program that provides health care services, Canada's health care system is a critical component of Canadian society, as much a national symbol as the maple leaf; the health care system serves as a "defining national characteristic distinguishing Canada from its neighbor to the south" (Jerome-Forget and Forget 1995). Although many admit their system is far from perfect, Canadians cherish their universal health care system and view it as one of government's success stories and a source of national pride.

Severe budget cutbacks resulting from a long-lasting recession[1] and an accompanying austerity program forced Canadian provinces to tighten their cost-control measures, significantly downsize the hospital sector, and

---

[1] The recession, which began in 1989, was technically over by 1991, although its aftershocks continued to be felt into the mid-1990s; for example, unemployment stood at 11.5 percent in 1993, and the Canadian economy did not register positive growth until 1996.

TABLE 6-1   Health Care in the United States and Canada

	United States	Canada
Life expectancy at birth, 1995	72.7 (male) 79.4 (female)	75.4 (male) 81.5 (female)
Median age of population, 1996	35	35
Projected percentage of population age 65 or older 2000 2010 2020	 12.5 13.6 17.5	 12.3 13.8 18.2
Health care expenditures, 1997 as % GDP per capita	 13.6 $4,090	 9.0 $2,095
Distribution of health care spending, 1997 (as percentage of total spending) Hospitals Physicians Pharmaceuticals	 34 20 8	 34 14 14
Physicians per 1,000 persons	2.6 (1996)	1.83 (1997)
Inpatient hospital beds per 1,000 persons, 1996	4.1	5.1 (1997)
Average length of stay (days), 1996	7.8	12
Scanners per million persons MRIs per million persons Lithotripters per million persons	26.9 (1993) 16 (1995) 1.5 (1990)	8.1 (1997) 1.7 (1997) 0.5 (1996)

Sources: OECD Health Data 98: A Comparative Analysis of 29 Countries, Paris: OECD/CREDES; World Bank; Canadian Institute for Health Information; Health Care Financing Administration.

curtail certain covered services. As the Canadian system completes its third full decade of operation, it faces problems in a number of areas, including lengthening waiting lists for medical services; insufficient long-term care services in the face of an aging population (Table 6–1); emergency room overcrowding; and lack of innovation in health care financing and delivery (OECD 1995). A growing share of overall health care expenditures now comes from the private sector, raising concerns about whether Canada's universal public system will gradually give way to a two-tiered system of coverage.

OVERVIEW OF CANADIAN HEALTH CARE

The Canadian health care system consists of twelve separate provincial and territorial plans[2] financed almost exclusively through public revenues in the form of a combination of provincial personal, sales, and corporate taxes and federal transfer payments. The provincial governments have jurisdiction over their health care systems; the federal government's role in health care is limited to specific groups,[3] accounting for less than 2 percent of total public health expenditure (OECD 1995).

Doctors are in private independent practices and are paid fees for their services. The majority of hospitals are operated by private, voluntary, nonprofit organizations. Despite the private delivery of services, the Canadian system features a high level of government regulation. Physicians' charges are fixed according to a negotiated fee schedule, and hospitals must operate within the parameters of a global budget, which also determines the availability of high technology medical equipment. Thus the Canadian system occupies a point toward the opposite end of the health care continuum from the U.S. system.

Although Canada's health care system is a blend of public finance and private delivery, the role of the private sector in Canadian health care has been deliberately limited. Canada's public insurance system covers all "medically required physician and hospital services" at no direct cost to the patient. Balance billing beyond the set fees is not allowed. Though individuals cannot purchase private insurance for services covered by the plans, the purchase of private insurance for services not covered by the plans is widespread.

Canadian health care expenditures, though significantly lower than those in the United States, grew at an annual rate of more than 10 percent between 1975 and 1991, and peaked at 10.2 percent of GDP in 1992. Rapidly rising costs combined with a serious economic recession forced provinces to tighten their fiscal belts and significantly curtail health care expenditures. Health care expenditures now represent 9.3 percent of GDP, the equivalent of their 1990 level. Canada, formerly the runner-up after the United States in terms of overall health care spending, has since ceded that place to Germany (Figure 6–1).

---

[2] The ten provinces and two territories are not homogenous; the provinces range from Ontario, where approximately one-third of the population resides, to the second largest province, French-speaking Quebec; to prosperous British Columbia and Alberta on the western side; the nation's breadbaskets Saskatchewan and Manitoba; the four relatively less prosperous provinces of New Brunswick, Newfoundland, Nova Scotia, and Prince Edward Island; and the two vast and sparsely populated territories, the Northwest and Yukon territories (White 1995).

[3] These include Native Canadians living on reserves, the military, the Royal Canadian Mounted Police, and inmates of federal penitentiaries (OECD 1994).

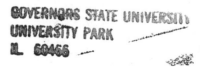

FIGURE 6-1   Health Care Expenditures, Canada, Germany, and the United States, 1970–1997 (as percentage of GDP)

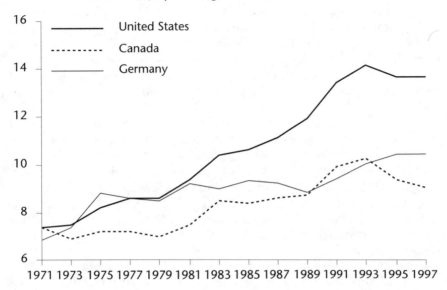

Source: OECD Health Data 98: A Comparative Analysis of 29 Countries. Paris: OECD/CREDES.

CANADIAN NATIONAL HEALTH INSURANCE: A LONG TIME COMING

The roots of Canada's most popular social program can be traced to the British North American Act of 1867, which laid out the parameters of responsibility for Canada's health care system. All aspects of the hospital sector—from construction and maintenance of facilities to all medical care provided within hospitals—were to fall within the purview of provincial governments. The federal government was to be responsible for such groups as Native Indians, Eskimos, and military personnel, as well as for food and drug legislation (Evans 1975).

The concept of a publicly financed health insurance program in Canada was first introduced in 1919, but it took the combined hardships of the Great Depression and World War II to bring national health insurance to the top of the legislative agenda. In the mid-1940s, public support for universal health care was strong. A 1944 Gallup poll revealed that 80 percent of the Canadian population was in favor of federally supported health insurance plans for each province. More important, as Malcolm Taylor, a preeminent historian on Canadian health care, pointed out, the public was willing to shoulder the cost of a national health plan (M. Taylor 1986). The concept also had the support of the Canadian Medical Association (CMA), although the medical profession demanded representation on all public health insurance commissions and final say over compensation methods (Andreopoulous 1975; Stevenson, Williams, and Vayda 1988).

Drawing on such broad-based public support, the federal government, as an enticement to encourage each of the provinces to set up provincial health insurance plans, offered to contribute funds to help defray some of the cost of health services. In return for these federal funds, the provinces had to turn over all personal and corporate income taxes to the federal government. This requirement proved to be too bitter a pill for the provinces to swallow, and the federal proposals were abandoned in 1945 (M. Taylor 1986).

Blue Cross, Blue Shield, and commercial insurance plans filled the void left by the unsuccessful attempt to set up a nationwide system of provincial health insurance plans. The development of these insurance plans eroded the initial base of support for a comprehensive national health insurance system, as medical, hospital, and insurance groups developed their own power bases. The CMA, meanwhile, shifted its position from support of public insurance to opposition; the collapse of federal proposals allowed the medical profession to create their own physician-controlled health insurance plans. These plans took hold in all the provinces (Stevenson et al. 1988). At the same time, however, federal–provincial relations— which had been strained by conflict over the initial proposals—gradually began to relax, and a consensus in support of national health insurance reemerged among provincial leaders (M. Taylor 1986).

HOSPITAL INSURANCE

The initial federal proposals were brought back to life when the province of Saskatchewan introduced a hospital insurance program in 1947. British Columbia followed suit in 1949, as did Alberta in 1950. When Newfoundland became part of Canada in 1949, approximately half its population was already covered by government hospital insurance. Thus even though attempts to create a national health insurance program had failed five years earlier, four Canadian provinces had functioning public hospital insurance plans by 1950.

The "demonstration effect" of these provincial programs was significant (Tuohy 1986). In 1957 the federal government passed the Hospital Insurance and Diagnostic Services Act, which served as the basis for a universal system of hospital insurance. Each province would receive federal grants that were to cover approximately half of the program's total cost. It is important to note that this was not a smooth, quick process; it took at least a decade for the federal and provincial governments to settle all the financial and administrative details (Anderson 1989).

While the plans were being formalized on the provincial level, concern arose that Canada might allow plans to develop in the provinces without federal oversight to ensure equity and regulate a standard level of benefits (Anderson 1989, 63). The granting of federal funds was made contingent on four conditions. First, each provincial plan had to be *comprehensive*, providing all medically necessary services with no benefits limitations. Second, plans had to be *publicly* administered on a nonprofit basis by a public agency accountable to the provincial government. Third, plan benefits had to be *universal*—available to all—and provided on uniform terms and conditions. Fourth, the interprovincial *portability* of plan benefits had to be ensured so that Canadians traveling outside their province of residence would still be covered.

As long as these four conditions were met, the federal government would allocate funds to contribute to the costs of the provincial hospital plans. This method of cost sharing ensured a nationwide standard of health care. Residents of such poorer provinces as Newfoundland would have access to the same standard of health care as those in such wealthier provinces as Ontario. Even though the provinces had to cede a certain amount of autonomy to the federal government in terms of control over the provincial plans, the cost-sharing offer was too good to refuse. By 1961 all ten provinces had hospital insurance plans that fulfilled the four criteria (M. Taylor 1986). These plans were very similar—if not duplicates of—the Blue Cross plans that were already in existence. In Ontario, for example, the government bought out Blue Cross's buildings, computer systems, and employees (Norton 1998).

The establishment of *hospital insurance plans* did not mean that the government took over the hospitals, however. Canadian hospitals remained voluntary, not-for-profit organizations under the direction of a board of trustees. What changed was the system of reimbursement: Provincial governments became the sole payers of hospital services (Barer 1988).

MEDICAL CARE INSURANCE

The success of the hospital program generated public support for an expansion to include medical care provided in areas other than hospitals (in other words, physicians' services). A Royal Commission appointed by the federal government in the early 1960s recommended the creation of a program to provide a wide range of medical benefits, partially supported by federal subsidies and administered by the provinces.

The medical care insurance program was not universally welcomed. In fact, it met large-scale opposition from the medical profession, the private insurance industry, and even several provincial governments. To win over the physicians, the federal government had to make certain assurances to the medical profession that their professional freedom would not be jeopardized by government intervention in the health care sector (Rachlis and Kushner 1989). But professional autonomy was not all the doctors were concerned about; there were more than ten private insurance plans controlled by physicians that covered four million people, and "business was booming" (Regush 1987, 28). The government assured the doctors (and tempered their opposition somewhat in the process) that the fee-for-service payment system and the system of fee schedules that existed in the physician-controlled insurance plans would be preserved.

The federal government pushed its program through despite the opposition of physicians and insurance groups, and the Medical Care Act went into effect in 1968. The same four conditions applying to the hospital plans governed disbursement of federal funds for physicians' services. Physician opposition declined as it became apparent that physicians would benefit financially from the new system; the doctors were less likely to complain in the face of "windfall professional income gains" as a result of payment basically being guaranteed by the new provincial plans (Stevenson et al. 1988, 69). As with the hospital insurance plans, these new physician plans were carbon copies of existing plans; in Ontario, for example, as it did with Blue Cross, the government essentially bought out the buildings, systems, and employees of Blue Shield (Norton 1998).

MEDICARE IS BORN

All ten provinces had full physician and hospital coverage by 1971, and the Yukon and Northwest territories followed a year later. Canada finally had a national health insurance program—known as Medicare—in place more than fifty years after the idea was first conceived. Nearly all hospital and physician services are covered under the plans, and all legal residents receive health care that is free at the point of service (although not "free" in the financial sense, as residents pay taxes that fund health care services; Lomas et al. 1989, 82). A critical principle guiding the Canadian health care system's formation was the removal of financial barriers to care. Another key feature of the system was the preservation of the freedom of choice for both patients and physicians: Patients remained free to choose their own physicians and hospitals, and physicians were free to choose where they wanted to practice.

The Canadian system of universal, comprehensive health care is rooted in the deeply held conviction that health care is a right, not a privilege. This conviction is illustrated by this statement by the Royal Commission: "What we seek is a method that will provide everyone in Canada with comprehensive coverage regardless of age, state of health, or ability to pay, upon uniform terms and conditions" (K. Brown 1989, 213).

Preventing a two-tier system of health care made up of those who could pay and those who could not was a high priority. The federal government determined that the best way to avoid such a two-tier system was to take the dramatic step of outlawing private insurance coverage for any services covered under the provincial plans. Provincial universal hospital and medical plans thus took the place of all the various forms of insurance—private, not-for-profit, and public—that had existed up to that point. The provincial governments became the single purchasers of publicly insured hospital and medical care services (M. Taylor 1986).

The advent of the Canadian provincial health insurance plans brought about a shift in financing from private to public channels. Consider, for example, that in 1960 more than one-third of the population had private comprehensive health insurance, and only 14 percent of expenditures for medical care came from public funding. By the mid-1970s, 95 percent of all costs of hospital and medical care services were paid through the provincial health plans and 0 percent of the population had private comprehensive health insurance coverage (Evans 1984).

The federal government, as discussed previously, was not granted constitutional authority to set up and manage a national health system. As a consequence, the health system that exists in Canada is actually a federal–provincial system that is a patchwork of separate provincial and territorial plans (Evans 1988b). The provinces are free to determine how their health care plans will be organized and their health care dollars spent. This is a crucial point, for, as Evans noted, "the division of powers between the federal government in Ottawa and the 10 provincial governments is Canada's longest and most carefully defended border" (Evans 1975, 129). At the same time, the federal government imposes certain regulations that tie the plans together.

The challenge of tying together ten provinces and two territories with diverse cultural and even legal systems should not be underestimated. Take Quebec—whose ongoing efforts to create an independent French-speaking region threaten to split the Canadian federation—as one example. More than one quarter of the Canadian population is of French origin; the province of Quebec not only has different cultural origins but a different legal system as well, based not on British common law as in the rest of the Canadian provinces, but on the Napoleonic Code.

POLITICAL AND CULTURAL UNDERPINNINGS OF CANADIAN HEALTH CARE

Social institutions such as health care systems are not created in a vacuum; they are reflections of societal values and expectations. Appreciation of the political and cultural environment in which the Canadian health care system evolved is essential to an understanding of the system itself and how resources are allocated and costs controlled. All legal residents of Canada are eligible for coverage under the provincial health insurance plans, and Canada thus does not have a significant portion of its population uninsured as the United States does. This difference highlights what one observer called the "remarkable egalitarian quality about Canadian health care that reflects a society that attaches a higher value to social equity than does the United States" (Iglehart 1986b, 781).

The Canadian and American political cultures share similar features: Both are multiparty systems based on democratic ideals. Both are also federal systems with state (province) and local-level government participation in public policy matters (Tuohy 1986). Despite these similarities, distinct features of each political culture have had a significant impact on the creation of each nation's social programs, particularly their health care systems.

One important feature—as noted by political theorist Louis Hartz—is that societies such as the United States, English Canada, French Canada, and Australia are "fragments," or offshoots, of European countries that developed independently in non-European lands. Despite shared British origins, the United States and English Canadian societies and their institutions evolved differently. Most notably, the American war of independence buried all vestiges of "tory" origins in the United States, and the "loyalists" in Canada kept their "tory touch" (Tuohy 1986, 396).

Yet in Canada this tory strain did not predominate. Instead, a rather strange mixture evolved, one containing remnants of the British tory conservatives combined with socialism. A socialist party was able to establish itself in Canada because its ideas did not differ significantly from the prevailing beliefs in society. Socialism in Canada, in the words of political theorist Gad Horowitz, "is British, non-Marxist and worldly," in contrast to the U.S. view of socialism as "German, Marxist, and other-worldly" (Tuohy 1986, 396).

Canada's distinctive political culture, known as *collectivism,* can be viewed as a combination of "capitalism with social responsibility—a kind of liberal conservatism or vice versa" (B. Brown 1989, 28). According to one analyst, Canada's collectivist culture "encourages a collaboration between the leadership of corporate groups and the state in the pursuit of redistributive policies" (Tuohy 1986, 396). The implications of this particular type of political culture are significant for the development of social programs:

> The coexistence of these elements has produced distinctive hybrids: "tory touched" liberals less distrustful of concentrated power than their U.S. counterparts; "red tories" supportive of redistributive policies implemented through public and private hierarchies; and democratic socialists willing

to pursue collectivist goals through the institutions of the state. (Tuohy 1986, 398)

The existence of this collectivist culture is central to the evolution of a health care system in Canada far different from its American counterpart. Canada's parliamentary system is a product of this political culture and thus focuses on consensus building. Such consensus building is not a feature of the U.S. system, whose diffuse bicameral political structure makes conflict the rule rather than the exception. Indeed, U.S. governmental institutions were created to check and balance power, in part, through the use of vetoes; the Canadian system does not contain such mechanisms (Tuohy 1986).

The inherent distrust of government on the part of many Americans leads to the search for "mechanistic, self-enforcing, automatic solutions" as a way of avoiding government intervention. The U.S. reliance on market forces in the health care sector can be understood in this context (Morone 1990, 133). Canadians, in contrast, have shown a greater willingness than Americans to grant government the key powers to finance and regulate health care programs (Lomas et al. 1989). Canada places a strong emphasis on using the government as a vehicle to attain goals consistent with the collective good. As Evans noted, "In Canada . . . the natural focus for collective activity has always been government. As residents of a small country . . . Canadians have instinctively turned to the state as the instrument of collective purposes" (Evans 1988b, 169).

The distinction comes into focus in the contrasting objectives spelled out in the constitutions of the United States and Canada. Life, liberty, and the pursuit of happiness are the stated goals in the United States; peace, order, and good government are the stated goals in Canada (Linton 1990b). The emphasis of the collective good over the individual shapes Canadian health care policy, particularly the Canadian approach to the distribution of scarce health care resources. Resources are allocated on the basis of need, not on the patient's financial standing, as " 'equality before the health care system' has been established as a . . . principle similar to 'equality before the law' " (Evans 1988b, 165). With this distinction and others in mind, let us now take a closer look at the Canadian system, how it operates, and how it differs from its U.S. counterpart.

HEALTH CARE DELIVERY IN CANADA

Health care in Canada is financed through tax revenues, with provincial governments playing a key role as the primary bill payers within the system. Canada's system is consequently often equated with "socialized medicine," similar to the system provided by Britain's state-owned National

Health Service. In fact, health care in Canada is provided through a private delivery system: Patients have free choice of physician, physicians are in private practice, and they are paid fees for the services they provide. This combination of public financing and private delivery can be described as socialized insurance. And though the Canadian system is referred to as national health insurance because the principles were set in law at the national, or federal, level, the management and delivery and to a large extent financing of health care are under the purview of each provincial or territorial government.

Coverage under the Plans

When Canadians need medical care, they go to the doctors of their choice and present their health cards. Patients do not fill out any forms, nor are they required to meet any deductible limits nor pay any copayments for medically necessary services (Health Canada 1997).

The federal legislation governing provincial health plans mandates that all medically necessary hospital and physician services are to be covered. Yet the concept of *medically necessary* has never been defined either by federal policy or legislation (Charles et al. 1997). As a result, the range of health care services provided by the provincial plans varies significantly across provinces, particularly in terms of prescription drug coverage, nursing home, and other long-term care, as well as services such as podiatry, physical therapy, chiropractic treatments, vision, and dental care. For instance, although seven provinces provide vision care coverage, all but two restrict coverage to children and those aged 65 and older. Likewise, though dental care in a hospital is covered by the provincial plans, out-of-hospital dental coverage is provided in five provinces and is limited to children, seniors, and individuals in income assistance programs.

Although all prescription drugs provided during a hospital stay are covered, no province has a universal drug plan that covers all out-of-hospital prescription drug costs for all residents, all but one of the provinces provide prescription drug plans for those aged 65 and older and those on income assistance programs. Three provinces have plans that provide coverage to all residents with copayments or deductibles (Buske 1998). And these can be substantial; for example, the annual family deductible was recently increased from CD $600 to $800[4] (for nonseniors) under the province of British Columbia's comprehensive pharmacare coverage plan (National Forum on Health 1997). The province of Quebec has a mandated universal prescription drug plan. All employers that provide

---

[4] As of June 1, 1998, CD $1.00 = U.S. $0.68.

health coverage to their active and retired employees must provide prescription drug coverage that is at least as generous as the government plan (Watson Wyatt 1997).

Long-term care services are provided to varying degrees and copayment requirements as a result of the Extended Health Care Services Program passed in 1977. Such services include health care, personal care, and social services provided in nursing homes or in the community. The individual's inability to function without the services is the criterion used to determine eligibility for nursing homes; the individual's income does not affect his or her eligibility status (Kane and Kane 1985).

The combination of escalating costs and budgetary pressures have led certain provinces to attempt to scale back the scope of covered services by deeming certain services not medically necessary and therefore eligible to be deinsured or removed from the list of covered services. These "delisted" services include tattoo removal, cosmetic surgery, and in-vitro fertilization, to name just a few. Most provinces have significantly cut back the amount they will pay for out-of-country coverage.

HOSPITALS

Nearly all of Canada's hospitals operate as private, nonprofit entities run by community boards of trustees, voluntary organizations, or municipalities. There are very few for-profit hospitals in Canada: Fewer than 5 percent of all hospitals are privately owned, and most of these are in the long-term care sector or provide such specialized services as addiction treatment (OECD 1995).

The number of hospital beds has declined significantly over the past decade as a result of efforts to control costs by shifting the focus of care from inpatient to less expensive outpatient services. Moreover, in light of the aging of the population, attention has turned to increasing the number of long-term care beds in an effort to free up acute care beds. For example, according to the Ontario Hospital Association, one out of ten beds in the average Toronto hospital is occupied by a patient ready to be discharged but with nowhere to go. More than half of these patients, known as "bed blockers," are in need of long-term care (Coutts 1998). Ontario recently introduced plans to expand the number of long-term care beds by 20,000 over an eight-year period (Spencer and Associates 1998).

Hospitals are funded primarily by the provincial health plans. The hospitals negotiate an annual lump-sum budget each year with the provincial health ministry or regional health authority. The hospital administrators then divide up the pie among the various departments (White 1995). The budgeting process serves to control the availability of high technology equipment, because the provincial government must approve all such purchases.

PHYSICIANS

The majority of doctors in Canada are in private practice, generally solo practice. Based on inaccurate assumptions about population growth, increases in the supply of physicians significantly outpaced population growth throughout the 1970s and 1980s. Provincial physician supply management measures have since slowed the increase, and the physician to population ratio dropped from 2.2 physicians per 1,000 population in 1993 to 1.83 in 1997.

Primary care is well-established in Canada; general practitioners and family practitioners represent 51 percent of all physicians and serve as the initial point of contact for patients, controlling access to most specialists and hospital admissions. Patients are free to choose their own primary care doctor, as well as certain specialists, including pediatricians, obstetricians, and ophthalmologists (Health Canada 1997; Mullan 1998).

Most physicians are paid on a fee-for-service basis. Doctors do not bill patients directly; rather they file a claim with the provincial health plan and are paid according to a fee schedule determined through negotiations between the provincial governments and the medical associations. Though physicians have the right to bill patients directly, essentially opting out of the provincial health system, very few do so. Except for dental surgery performed in a hospital, dentists practice outside the provincial health system (Health Canada 1997).

CANADIAN HEALTH CARE FINANCING

The Canadian provinces finance health care through a combination of provincial tax revenues and federal transfer funds. Some provinces draw on additional funding sources not specifically earmarked for health care, such as sales taxes, payroll taxes, and lottery proceeds, but these funds play a small role in overall health care financing. Two provinces (Alberta and British Columbia) charge health care premiums, but these are not risk-based premiums nor do they affect an individual's access to services. Those with low incomes receive assistance paying the premiums, and many employers cover the cost of the premiums for their employees. Although Canadian health care is essentially free at the point of service (patients never see a bill), it is by no means *free* to the individual. Individual income taxes and sales taxes are significantly higher in Canada than the United States.

FEDERAL FINANCING CHANGES: 1977, 1984, AND 1996

Health care financing in Canada has gone through three major changes over the past two decades. First, the enactment of the Federal–Provincial

Fiscal Arrangements and Established Programs Financing Act (EPF) in 1977 effectively instituted a cap on the federal contribution to provincial health plans. Second, the passage of the Canada Health Act in 1984 ushered in one of the more controversial periods in the history of Canadian health care by pitting the medical profession against the public. Third, the introduction of the Canadian Health and Social Transfer in 1996 again changed the way the federal government transfers health care funds to the provinces.

THE EPF By the mid-1970s the Canadian federal government had become concerned about rising health care expenditures. Although the federal government matched all provincial expenditures, it had no control over total expenditures. For their part, the provinces were not overly concerned with holding down costs because they were spending "50-cent dollars"; they knew whatever amount they spent would be matched by federal funds (M. Taylor 1986).

The federal government rectified this situation by retreating from its open-ended commitment to fund provincial health plans, enacting the EPF in 1977. This law set out a new method of cost-sharing in which the government traded its prior arrangement of matching provincial health costs on a 50–50 basis for a system of per capita health care payments in the form of block grants (which included funds for postsecondary education as well as health care). In return, a certain amount of personal and corporate income tax revenue was to be shifted to the provinces. This new financing scheme tied increases in federal financial support for provincial health plans to economic growth measured by increases in GNP. The provinces would therefore be bound to cover a larger share of the health care costs when these costs increased faster than the nation's overall economic growth (Iglehart 1986b). In this way, the federal government could use the cap on federal funds to foster cost control at the provincial level.

Though the EPF shifted the responsibility for cost control to the provinces, the federal government maintained a measure of control over the system, because disbursement of the block grants was linked to compliance with national standards. Federal funds were contingent on fulfilling the four criteria (comprehensiveness, public administration, universality, and portability) outlined earlier.

The EPF was a watershed in the development of the Canadian health care system for two reasons. First, it "represented the most massive transfer in history of revenues (and therefore of the substance of power) from the federal to the provincial governments" (M. Taylor 1986, 25). Second, it completely changed the ratio of federal–provincial funds for health care. From 1977 on, the annual rate of health cost increases would have to stay in line with GNP increases, with the provinces on the hook for any excess amount.

The federal government tinkered with the formula throughout the 1980s in an effort to limit the growth of EPF transfers. For example, in

1986 the formula was revised to link EPF increases to GNP growth less 2 percent. In 1990 the Expenditure Control Plan froze entitlement levels for a period of five years.

The ultimate result of the EPF legislation has been a significant increase in the provincial share of health care costs, as the growth of health care costs consistently outpaced that of economic growth. In 1980 the federal government covered nearly one-third of provincial health care expenditures; ten years later the federal share had dropped to less than one quarter. Current figures put the federal share at 21.5 percent. An average of one-third of all provincial budgets now goes to fund health care services, up from approximately 28 percent in 1980 (Marshall 1998).

THE CANADA HEALTH ACT OF 1984. The second major piece of legislation with important financial implications for Canadian health care was the Canada Health Act of 1984. The Act was partly a consequence of a series of wage and price controls implemented by the federal government during an inflationary period in the mid-1970s. When the government relaxed these controls, physicians used the vehicle of balance billing—that is, charging more than the fee schedule would allow—to make up for the previous period of austerity. This practice was seen to be in direct conflict with the philosophical core of Canadian health care: Equal access for all. A commission created by the federal government to study this issue found that balance billing (or extra billing, as it is sometimes called) was indeed compromising access to care for those unable to pay the extra fees (M. Taylor 1986).

According to health economist Morris Barer, then-prime minister Pierre Elliott Trudeau, with his reelection hanging in the balance, seized on the issue as a political life raft and proposed the Canada Health Act (Barer 1988; Iglehart 1986b). The act made extra billing by physicians illegal. The medical profession opposed the act on the grounds that extra billing was a safety valve offering protection from the powerful provincial governments that set physicians' fees. Provincial governments opposed the bill on the grounds that it infringed on their constitutional rights (Iglehart 1986b). Whereas the EPF transferred power to the provinces, the Canada Health Act was considered an "unwarranted and powerful federal intrusion into a field of provincial jurisdiction" by the provincial government and the medical associations (M. Taylor 1986, 25).

The Canada Health Act enjoyed tremendous public support, and no government official with any survival instinct would vote against it. The bill breezed through Parliament unopposed, despite strong opposition from the medical profession and provincial governments. The act imposed a strict penalty on those provinces that permitted extra billing: Federal grants would be reduced in direct proportion to the extra billing charges. In other words, for every dollar charged directly to a patient, the province would lose one dollar in federal funds.

The reaction to the passage of the Canada Health Act was particularly heated in Ontario, where the Ontario Medical Association challenged the legality of the bill and called a strike to put pressure on the provincial government to repeal it. The strike, the longest in Canadian history, was called off after twenty-five days. The conflict over extra billing "drew sharp lines of battle between the majority of the physicians in the country and the majority of the population. The population won" (Evans 1988b, 168). The CHA essentially reaffirmed the commitment to Medicare's original four core principles and added the fifth principle of accessibility—that the provincial plan must provide access to covered services without financial barriers. All ten provinces had passed legislation by 1987 to ban extra billing. However, the deep rifts that developed between the provincial health care payers and providers over the extra billing issue continue to this day.

1996 FINANCING CHANGE. The federal government enacted a third change to the way it finances health care in 1996 with the introduction of the Canadian Health and Social Transfer (CHST). The CHST combines federal contributions for health care, welfare, and postsecondary education into a new single block transfer, which is essentially a combination of cash contributions and tax points. The CHST replaced the EPF block transfers; as in the past, the provinces must adhere to the principles of the Canada Health Act to receive full federal transfer payments (Embassy of Canada 1997; Marshall 1998).

THE PRIVATE SIDE OF HEALTH CARE FINANCING

Concurrent with the increasing financial burden borne by the provinces in the wake of declining federal contributions, there has been an increase in the share of total health care paid by private sources. Private sources include employer-sponsored plans, individual supplemental health insurance plans, and out-of-pocket expenditures. The private share surpassed 30 percent of all health care expenditures in 1997 (Figure 6–2).

The rising share of expenditures covered by private sources is driven by rapidly rising pharmaceutical drug costs as well as provincial limits on certain services—the delisting of laser and cosmetic surgery, for example, has fueled the growth of private clinics providing such services. Government coverage of out-of-country medical services has been sharply curtailed, and these costs have been shifted to the private sector. In 1995, for example, the government of Ontario sharply curtailed payments for medical services provided outside Canada, shifting from an open-ended fee-for-service reimbursement to a flat per diem rate of CD $400 for emergency hospital care (Katz, Verrilli, and Barer 1998).

The rapid rise in costs paid for by private funds stands in stark contrast to the growth in costs for public sector care. Whereas the annual in-

FIGURE 6-2   The Growing Private Sector Share of Health Spending 1991–1998
(as percentage of total health care spending)

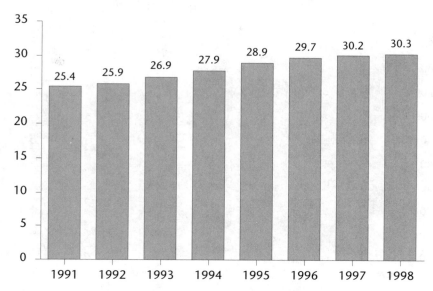

Source: Canadian Institute for Health Information, 1998, "National Health Expenditure Trends, 1975–1998."

crease in public health expenditures has been flat or negative over the past few years, annual increases in private health spending has consistently surpassed 5 percent (Health Canada 1997).

A large share of private health care expenditures are paid for by employers who contribute to the health care costs of their employees in many ways: through the payment of corporate taxes, contributions to Workmen's Compensation boards in the majority of the provinces, health insurance premiums in the provinces that levy such charges, and through supplemental health benefit programs.

Though federal law prohibits private health insurance companies from covering medical services that fall within the scope of the provincial health plans, supplemental health insurance plans are widely available to cover medical costs for services such as dental and vision care, prescription drugs, semiprivate and private hospital rooms not covered by the plans. According to the Canadian Life and Health Insurance Association, 20.6 million Canadians had supplemental coverage in 1997,[5] up from 18

---

[5] The number of Canadians insured for supplemental or extended health care was 13.5 million, and an additional 7.1 million were insured for dental care.

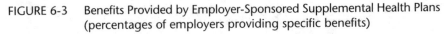

FIGURE 6-3   Benefits Provided by Employer-Sponsored Supplemental Health Plans
(percentages of employers providing specific benefits)

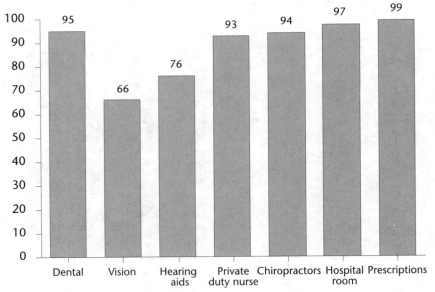

Source: The Wyatt Company 1993 Survey of Group Benefits Plans Covering Salaried Employees
of Canadian Employers.

million ten years earlier. Employer contributions for supplemental health
insurance are tax deductible and not considered a taxable benefit to employees in any of the provinces except Quebec (Watson Wyatt 1997).

A 1993 survey of nearly 1,000 Canadian companies revealed that
most employers sponsor a supplemental health benefit plan providing private hospital room and prescription drug coverage, and 95 percent provide
dental benefits (Figure 6–3). The survey found that 28 and 30 percent of
employers, respectively, require the employee to contribute toward the
premium cost for single and family coverage (Wyatt Company 1993).

In addition to the shift in the financing burden from the federal to the
provincial governments and the growing share of private sources in overall health care financing, one final financing change bears note: A significant change has occurred in the way health care dollars are spent. As
noted earlier, the provinces, in a determined effort to control costs, implemented a shift in focus away from institutional care to community-
based ambulatory care, focusing resources on less expensive outpatient
and clinic settings. Funding for hospitals dropped from nearly 41 percent
of total health care spending in 1987 to less than 34 percent in 1997 (Figure 6–4). A decade of downsizing in the hospital sector has resulted in a

FIGURE 6-4   Where the (Canadian) Dollars Go: Health Expenditures by Sector, 1987 and 1997 (as percentages of total health care spending)

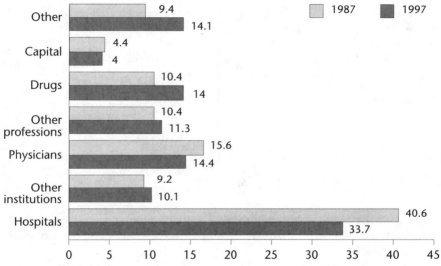

Source: Canadian Institute for Health Information, "National Health Expenditure Trends, 1975–1998."

Note: 1997 data are estimated.

20 percent reduction in the number of hospital beds across Canada (Marshall 1998).

Over the period from 1986 to 1996, outpatient medical services increased nearly 70 percent, and outpatient surgery increased 34 percent. In contrast, the use of emergency room services declined by 17 percent over the same time period (Marshall 1998).[6]

Expenditures on drugs have risen significantly over the past decade, to the point where the National Forum on Health, a federal advisory body charged with evaluating the future direction of the Canadian health care system, recommended in February 1997 that a national single-payer system for pharmaceutical drugs be introduced. The forum reasoned that pharmaceutical drugs fall within the definition of medically necessary ser-

---

[6] Despite the decline in the overall use of emergency room services, serious overcrowding in most hospital emergency rooms remains a persistent problem. This is a result, in part, to the fact that physicians still practice in solo or small group practices (one to three doctors); if a patient calls a doctor past 4:30 P.M. they are likely to get a recorded message to go to the emergency room for treatment. I am grateful to my colleague Jim Norton for pointing this out to me.

TABLE 6-2   Prescription Drugs: Who's Covered, Who Pays?

Prescription drug coverage (by type of coverage)	Percentage of population	Drug expenditures (by source of payment)	Percentage of total drug expenditures
Provincial plans	44	Provincial plan	44
Private plans	44	Private plans	28
Uninsured	12	Individuals (copayments, deductibles, and out-of-pocket payments)	28

Source: National Pharmacare Cost Impact Study 1997.

vices and therefore all Canadians should be guaranteed coverage against the rising costs of drugs, and that a single-payer system could more effectively control costs.

Currently slightly more than one-tenth of the population has no coverage against the cost of prescription drugs (Table 6–2). Yet even those with coverage face significant costs given that both public and private plans typically require copayments and impose deductible limits. These limits can be sufficiently high as to make it unlikely that an individual will receive any reimbursement for drug expenditures.

The provinces, through their pharmacare programs, shoulder the cost of 44 percent of all drug expenditures, with the remainder covered by employers through private insurance plans and individuals through copayments, deductibles, and out-of pocket payments (Dingwall 1997; National Pharmacare Cost Impact Study 1997).

HEALTH CARE COST-CONTROL, CANADIAN-STYLE

In contrast to the U.S. multipayer health care system, the Canadian provincial governments are the sole payers for publicly insured services. Health economist Robert Evans has made the analogy between Canadian cost-control processes and a U.S. HMO: "In a sense, our provincial plans are super HMOs, each with a geographical monopoly, negotiating with a fractious group of providers, and under political rather than market constraints to keep costs down" (Evans 1986a, 34). Provincial governments use their monopsony (sole purchaser) power to control the two largest sources of health care expenditures: hospitals and physicians services, which together account for nearly half of all health care spending.

HOSPITALS

Tight controls on hospital budgets are critical to overall cost control because the hospital sector consumes the largest share of provincial health care budgets. Hospital operating expenses are kept separate from funds for capital expenditures. Annual global (total) hospital budgets for operating expenses are negotiated between the provincial governments and each individual hospital. In Ontario, for example, hospitals are given an annual global budget (in the form of a lump-sum payment) by the Ministry of Health that "serves as a fiscal envelope within which each hospital must function for the following year" (Naylor 1991, 111).

Each hospital is then responsible for allocating resources for all the different hospital services from its one budget. Annual budgets are not usage-sensitive. It does not matter if a patient comes in for a coronary bypass operation or to seek care for a sprained ankle: All costs are applied against the hospital's overall budget. A hospital will budget, for example, for a certain number of elective coronary artery bypass surgical procedures. If more than the predetermined number of patients need the procedure, a waiting list is created and patients are ranked according to need.

The separation of operating expenses from capital expenditures enables the provinces to exert control over increasing capacity, and ultimately over total hospital expenditures. All new capital expenditures to build new facilities, renovate existing facilities, or procure major pieces of medical equipment must be approved in advance by the provincial ministry of health. Although hospitals can raise capital from independent sources for new facilities or equipment, government approval is needed to use provincial plans to cover the operating expenses of the new facility or procedure. In other words, a hospital might be able to raise enough money to purchase a magnetic resonance imager (MRI), but the hospital would need the provincial ministry's permission for funds necessary to operate the machine.

Most major advanced technologies are concentrated in hospitals. For example, all computerized tomography (CT) scanners are in hospitals (enforced by law in Ontario). This concentration of high technology services in hospitals, and the control over hospital budgets by provincial governments, slows the diffusion of technology. For example, the United States has three times as many CAT scanners per million people as Canada, and more than ten times as many MRIs. The technology control inherent in Canada's highly centralized budgeting process is an integral component of the system's overall cost control strategy. Yet limits on medical technology force physicians to prioritize treatment on the basis of need, which translates into significant waiting times for certain procedures, as described further later in the chapter. Moreover, global budgets do not allow the provinces the flexibility to respond to changing patterns of demand for health care services. Hospital budgets are determined by past utilization, with little focus on future health care needs (OECD 1995).

The cutbacks in health care funding that have been the hallmark of the 1990s have resulted in hospital budgets being frozen or reduced. Hospital administrators have been forced to look to innovative approaches to management and overall organizational structure in the face of the new, less kind fiscal environment.

PHYSICIANS' EXPENDITURES

The second largest health care expenditure category is physicians' services. Unlike the hospital sector, the physician expenditure category was, up until the late 1980s, relatively open-ended: Although physicians' services were priced according to a fee schedule, there was no control over the volume of services provided. Rising costs forced the provinces to tighten their cost-control measures, and the battle to control physician expenditures has been waged on several fronts: physicians fees, utilization levels, and physician supply.

PHYSICIANS' FEES. Doctors in Canada are paid directly from the provincial budgets on a fee-for-service basis according to a fee schedule that establishes a price for each medical service. The total percentage increase in the fee base is hammered out during negotiations between the provincial ministries of health and the provincial medical associations. The provincial medical association then determines how the increase will be divided among the different medical specialties and services.

The negotiating process has evolved over time. The transition from physician-controlled plans to the establishment of provincial insurance plans with the government as major paymaster markedly altered the structure of fee negotiations and caused a shift in the balance of power between the health care providers (physicians) and payers (provincial governments). Barer shed light on this important transition:

> Whereas previously the physician-controlled insurance programs had essentially administered an orderly escalation of fees and incomes, under the new regime provincial governments had to bear the political costs of raising the necessary funds. Fee schedules were subsequently negotiated, not promulgated, and the negotiations became serious. (1988, 12)

Even in the early years of national health insurance, provincial governments tended to accept the medical associations' fee schedules and agreed to pay physicians 85 to 100 percent of the amounts set out in those schedules. Physicians agreed to less than full reimbursement because they would no longer have to be concerned with bad debts—patients not paying their bills—as the government would be the sole payer. As the system matured, however, formal negotiations replaced the province's nearly automatic acceptance of the medical associations' fee schedules (Lomas et al. 1989). The negotiations—once described as "large-scale political theater with all the rhetorical threats and flourishes that political clashes require"—are designed to determine the total percentage increase for physicians' services (Evans et al. 1989, 576).

Recent negotiations reveal the strong bargaining position of the provincial governments. Doctors contend that fee negotiations occur only in theory; in practice provincial governments impose their will on physicians because "in the end the provincial government can determine what fees it will pay on a 'take it or leave it' basis" (Barer 1988, 15). This is precisely what happened in Ontario during the 1989 fee schedule negotiations. The medical associations and the provincial government reached a stalemate in the negotiations. The government unilaterally imposed a 1.75 percent increase in the fee schedule, rejecting the physicians' demand for a higher increase (Linton 1990a). From 1990 to 1996, annual increases were limited to less than 1 percent. Such exercises of absolute control over fee schedules have resulted in a substantial amount of physician disaffection in Canada.

CONTROLLING UTILIZATION. By the late 1980s the provincial governments had come to realize that costs would continue to increase because fee schedules did not offer any way to control the utilization of services. The Canada Health Act effectively banned billing beyond the amount indicated on the physician fee schedule; given physicians are paid on a fee-for-service basis, one way for physicians to augment their incomes is to provide more services. Increases in utilization levels, combined with sluggish economic growth, prompted all of the provinces to implement mechanisms to control utilization by linking such increases to fee schedules (Lomas et al. 1989).

All ten provinces now impose caps on total physician expenditures, with the majority of the provinces using "hard caps," which essentially means that there is a fixed pot of money available for physicians' expenditures over a set period of time. Any amount beyond the cap must be reimbursed by physicians, generally through an adjustment in fee levels (Hurley, Lomas, and Goldsmith 1997).[7] Clearly, the level at which the cap is set is critical to its cost-control effectiveness. Some provinces base the amount on such factors as population growth and demographic changes, and others account for such factors as changes in physician supply, new technology, public-sector wage increases, and changes in practice overhead costs (Barer, Lomas and Sanmartin 1996).

---

[7] In contrast, under a "soft cap," also known as an expenditure target, both physicians and payers share the liability for excess expenditures (Hurley et al. 1997).

In addition to caps on total physician expenditures, five of the ten provinces have a cap on individual physicians' incomes as well. The process varies across the provinces, but as an example, in Ontario, once a physician has earned CD $404,000 in any fiscal year, the next $50,000 in fees are paid at 67 percent, and fees beyond that are paid at 33 percent (Barer et al. 1996).

Although there always has been significant conflict between the provinces and the physicians, expenditure and income caps have ratcheted this conflict to a higher level. In British Columbia, for example, physicians' payments were "clawed back" by 2.9 percent in 1997 and 4.4 percent in 1998. Physicians stopped working for three days in June 1998 to protest the yawning gap between the government-set expenditure cap and the services provided to patients (Lindsay 1998).

Increasing public demand for services continues to bump up against provincial attempts to hold down costs, and physicians are caught in the cross-fire; the government has put the physicians in the role of risk-bearing gatekeepers financially liable for expenditures that surpass the limit (Lindsay 1998). Despite this conflictual relationship between the provincial governments and the physicians, fewer than 1 percent of all physicians leave Canada—a rate that has held steady since the 1980s. Statistics recently released by the Canadian Institute for Health Information (CIHI) reveal that in 1997 the actual number of active civilian physicians that left Canada was 10 percent lower than in 1996.

PHYSICIAN SUPPLY. Not surprisingly, tight control over physician expenditures has led to efforts to control physician supply; expenditure caps introduce a "zero-sum" game in that new entrants to the profession represent more competitors for a slice of the income pie. This is particularly true if the cap does not factor in changes in physician supply.

Physician supply policies vary from province to province and do not represent a coordinated national approach to physician supply; policies include reduced fees on new physicians in three provinces (new physicians who do not have hospital privileges in Prince Edward Island, for example, are paid at a rate of 50 percent of fees) and restrictions on billing numbers in five provinces (physicians cannot be paid by the provincial plan without a billing number and the provinces use selective criteria to grant these numbers). In Ontario, physicians trained outside the province are not allowed to practice under the public plan; in Saskatchewan, foreign physicians are not allowed to practice under the public plan. In addition, many of the provinces have reduced their medical school enrollments (Barer et al. 1996).

As the previous discussion reveals, Canada has relied on a cost-control approach that attacks expenditures on several fronts: physicians' fees, overall physician expenditures, and physician supply. This integrated approach, along with the more blunt tool of direct budget cutbacks, has significantly slowed the rise in health care spending levels. Health care spending increases, which averaged 11 percent over the period between 1975 and 1991, fell to less than 3 percent a year between 1991 and 1995, and even further to 1.4 percent between 1995 and 1997. Cost control has not been a painfree process, however. Indeed, the impact of budget cutbacks combined with tight cost control measures is evident in significant waiting times for specific medical services.

The Canadian system's allocation of scarce resources according to need seems to be a logical means of preserving the universality of access given that "under circumstances of universal coverage, queueing is the most likely substitute for differential insurance status as a rationing mechanism" (Vladek 1986, 444). But such queueing, according to a report published by the Fraser Institute, a conservative think tank, is the clearest sign of the system's severe funding problems. The institute's report revealed that although there are significant variations in waiting times across the provinces, the average Canada-wide wait for treatment in 1997 was twelve weeks from referral by a GP to treatment by a specialist. The waiting time has increased from eleven weeks in 1996 and nine weeks in 1993. The waits for treatment tend to be the longest for elective cardiovascular surgery (eighteen weeks), orthopaedic surgery (twenty-one weeks) and ophthalmology (twenty-five weeks). In addition, the study found the median wait for an MRI was ten weeks and for a CT scan four weeks (Ramsay and Walker 1998).

Lengthy waits for certain procedures drive many Canadians to seek care across the border in the United States. A veritable cottage industry of firms dedicated to arranging timely treatment in the United States for Canadians who can afford to pay has developed (Kirkey 1997). Though the popular perception is that the extent of cross-border care is significant and growing, it is not clear how widespread the phenomenon actually is. One recent study of Ontario residents crossing the U.S. border to seek care concluded that although there certainly are people who go to the United States for certain services, "These occurrences represent a tip without an iceberg" (Katz et al. 1998).

The Canadian government, for its part, is concerned about a lack of quality data regarding waiting times and questions the accuracy of the Fraser Institute's findings. The government has announced it will use the Health Transition Fund to finance a national project called "From Chaos to Order: Making Sense of Waiting Lists in Canada." The project aims to develop a standardized source of data to track national information on waiting lists, and to use that information to develop an improved process to manage access to health services.

THE FUTURE OF CANADIAN HEALTH CARE

Shrinking resources are forcing Canada to look beyond the stringent cost-control measures to other avenues for getting the most out of its health care dollars; as Robert Evans pointed out, "The question of health care reform becomes one of trying to figure out how to do more with less" (Jerome-Forget, White, and Wiener 1995). The growing pressures on the Canadian health care system stem from the inherent difficulties in promising to be all things to all people: universal access not tied to ability to pay; comprehensive coverage; professional freedom for physicians and patient choice of provider, all the while controlling costs. The system may be reaching a critical point; polls indicate ebbing levels of public satisfaction: In 1990, 63 percent of Canadians rated the quality of health care as excellent or very good; only 37 percent currently do so (Sibbald 1998).

Health Care Devolution

One approach to improving the efficiency of the health care sector, and thereby "do more with less," has been the decentralization or devolution of a significant amount of authority over health care from the provincial to the regional and local levels in all provinces except Ontario. In Quebec, for example, the provincial health system was broken into eighteen separate regions, and each is overseen by a separate board of directors. These regional boards are responsible for the planning, coordination, financing, and evaluation of health care services in the province. In British Columbia, devolution has involved the formation of eighty-two community health councils reporting to twenty regional health boards. In Alberta seventeen regional health authorities have been created to replace more than 200 separate health boards and administrations. In Saskatchewan more than 400 single-function health boards have been replaced by thirty locally elected district health boards (U.S. and Foreign Commercial Service 1997).

Devolution is viewed not only as a way to control costs but also as a means to "improve health outcomes, increase the flexibility and responsiveness of care delivery and better integrate and coordinate services" (Lomas, Wood, and Veenstra 1997). Local health boards receive funding from provincial governments through global budgets and are responsible for planning, priority setting, allocating health funds, and managing services. The provinces have not ceded financial control for two of the three biggest expenditure categories, however. Physicians services and prescription drugs remain outside of the devolved budget (Lomas et al. 1997).

It is still too early to tell what the ultimate impact of devolution will be; indeed, the process of devolution is still ongoing in many provinces. One theory behind devolution is that shifting control over health care decisions to the regional or local level will shield health care decisions from powerful provincial political pressures; as a result it is hoped that decisions regarding the allocation of health care resources will be evidence-based rather than politically based. It is not yet clear, however, whether this theory will ultimately come to be realized in practice (Lomas 1997).

USER FEES

Constant struggles over appropriate levels of health care financing inevitably lead to discussions over the implementation of user fees. Such fees are considered by some to be a means of infusing added resources into the financially struggling health care system, as well as an effective way to reduce overconsumption, to raise individuals' awareness of the importance of health prevention measures, and to reduce unnecessary use of health services (OECD 1995).

All provinces charge some form of user fees (in the form of copayments for pharmaceutical drug coverage), but all medically necessary services are provided to patients at no extra charge as a core principle of the Canada Health Act. Indeed, fees over and above what Canadians pay in taxes are extremely controversial and raise fears of an erosion of universal access and the creation of a two-tiered system of coverage.

A 1997 survey revealed that more than half of all respondents supported the introduction of user fees, whereas 44 percent said the system should be financed completely by taxes. Nearly three quarters of respondents to a 1993 Angus Reid poll supported a proposed user fee of $5 for emergency room visits.

CONVERGENCE

Although there are no signs of the U.S. system moving toward the Canadian model of publicly financed universal health care, certain elements of U.S.-style managed care are beginning to appear in Canada. Although the appearance of tools of the managed care trade within employer-sponsored supplemental health plans may not be surprising, what is intriguing is the introduction of certain elements of managed care within the provincial health plans.

EMPLOYER PLANS TURN TO MANAGED CARE

Though Canadian employers pay less for their employee health benefit programs than their U.S. counterparts, the cost of employee benefit programs in Canada is significant and has risen considerably over the past decade. This is particularly true for prescription drugs, whose costs absorbs the lion's share of employer-sponsored benefits programs. Private sector expenditures on drugs more than doubled between 1984 and 1994.

Up until recently Canadian employers were basically in the same position that U.S. employers were in during the 1980s in terms of implementing strategies that shifted costs to employees and imposed restrictions on what benefit plans would cover (Norton 1998). Some Canadian employers are gradually turning to elements of U.S.-style managed care programs, with a particular focus on reining in rising drug expenditures. Managed drug care programs are relatively new and as a result are not yet used by a majority of employers, according to Watson Wyatt's 1996 Canadian Health/Dental Cost Management and Flexible Benefits survey. Programs that are being used by employers include formulary, or a recommended list of high-quality drugs, generic substitution, drug utilization review, preferred provider networks, and mail order services (Figure 6–5).

Mail order pharmacy took off in Canada in 1992, but by 1995 revenues represented less than 1 percent of all prescriptions. Though revenues are expected to grow to 5 percent by 2004, real expansion in mail order pharmacy faces significant obstacles, including the regulation of drug prices; the already high rates of generic substitution; and regulations governing the shipment of pharmaceuticals between provinces (*Medical & Healthcare Marketplace Guide* 1997).

Watson Wyatt's survey revealed that employer-sponsored managed drug programs are most prevalent in Ontario. And the province is taking further steps down the managed care road, with the introduction of a primary care reform program, which features rostering arrangements that are close cousins to physician networks in the United States and U.K. gatekeeper arrangements. The government hopes that individuals will choose to sign up (roster) with one physician, thus cutting back on the practice of going to several physicians for the same medical complaint, as well as use of emergency rooms for nonemergency care.

Approximately 200 doctors will participate in the program, and approximately 300,000 patients will have the opportunity to enroll with a family physician. Enrollment is voluntary; the government estimates that at least 75 percent of patients will enroll in the program. The program essentially involves a curtailment of patients' free choice of provider (once patients sign up they can only see that physician), but in return for signing up with a single physician patients will receive expanded access to on-call services, after-hours telephone nurse lines, and additional health prevention and education information.

Under the pilot program, individual doctors will group together in networks or large clinics to provide around-the-clock health services for enrolled patients. Funding from the Ministry of Health will be on a capi-

FIGURE 6-5   Managed Drug Care Programs, 1996 (by number of Canadian companies)

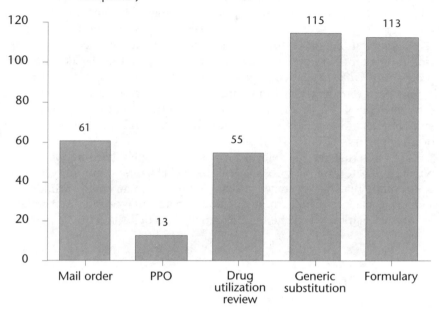

Source: Watson Wyatt 1996 Canadian Health/Dental Cost Management and Flexible Benefits Survey.

tation basis, according to the number, age, and gender of the physicians' enrolled patients. Ontario is no stranger to capitated funding arrangements, as there are seventy-seven health services organizations in the province that provide a range of primary care services to patients and are funded on a capitated basis. (Government of Ontario 1998; Morrison 1998; Schneider 1998).

It is not clear what the outcome of Ontario's experiment with rostering will be. But the mere existence of the pilot program puts Canada on a track similar to Germany in terms of the application of managed care techniques within the confines of a national health insurance system (Germany) and single-payer universal health care system (Canada).

INTERNAL MARKETS IN CANADIAN HEALTH CARE SYSTEM

Although it will be interesting to track the evolution and adaptation of managed care techniques in both the private and public sectors of Canadian health care, an additional sign of convergence between the Canadian and other health care systems lies in recent reform proposals that call for the creation of an internal market, similar to reform programs implemented in the Netherlands and the United Kingdom. Canada's version of the internal market would preserve the system's public funding but would rely on capitation and the use of gatekeepers—family physicians that control budgets for services (Jerome-Forget and Forget 1998). Like the pilot program in Ontario, patients would register with a family physician who would be the manager of funds provided by the government for patient care. Groups of physicians would form networks to not only provide services but also to purchase services from hospitals and specialists on behalf of their patients (Coutts 1998a).

The internal market reform proposals will likely become part of the ongoing debate over how to preserve the Canadian system's universal access, comprehensive coverage, and public funding in an era of shrinking resources. Canadians can learn much about the advantages and disadvantages of internal markets from the U.K. experience, as described in Chapter 7.

CHAPTER 7

Reforming the British National Health Service

Previous chapters have examined the health care systems of other nations that were once considered as potential models of reform for the U.S. health care system. Britain's National Health Service (NHS),[1] on the other hand, is often presented in the United States as precisely the opposite: something to avoid rather than emulate, an example of the negative consequences of government ownership and control of health care. For many Americans, the NHS is akin to "health care run by the Post Office" (R. Smith 1998), and descriptions of the NHS in the U.S. literature tend to be accompanied by accounts of rationing "designed to evoke horror and revulsion" and to underscore the unacceptability of a British-style system for the United States (Marmor and Klein 1986, 20).

Such views beg the question of why one should bother to study the British system at all. Although it is not likely that the United States would ever adopt the British model of health care, there are several very good reasons why the British system merits U.S. attention. First, the NHS was the pioneer of national health care. Whereas Bismarck's social insurance program blazed new trails in the field of legislating coverage for workers, the NHS set a precedent as the first comprehensive, nationalized system of health care as distinct from health insurance.

Second, the NHS is the largest, most centralized, public health care system in Europe, and with more than one million workers it is Europe's largest employer. The system treats more than 30 million patients annually, and had a budget of approximately $70 billion in 1998. Private insurance covers approximately 12 percent of the population but provides coverage for only a limited range of treatment. As such it is a supplement rather than a replacement for the NHS. Thus the entire British population depends on the NHS for most of its health care needs, and despite its many problems the NHS does an adequate job of keeping the population

---

[1] The description in this chapter is limited to England only, and as such does not focus on the other areas of the United Kingdom: Wales, Scotland, or Northern Ireland.

healthy when measured in terms of such indicators as life expectancy and infant mortality rates, which are similar to those in the United States.

Third, it is important to examine a system that represents for many Americans the epitome of "socialized medicine" and provides fuel for discussions supporting or opposing nationalized health care. To proponents of nationalized health care, the NHS represents an equitable and cost-effective approach to providing health care services. Critics of the NHS model, on the other hand, focus on its weaknesses, particularly the pervasive funding problems, and the most visible sign of the system's problems: long waiting lists for certain forms of medical treatment.

The profound differences between the way the United States and Britain finance and provide health care for their populations reflect significant political, cultural, and economic differences between the two nations. Although the United States and Britain share a common language, commitment to democratic ideals, and similar medical education systems (Aaron and Schwartz 1990), Britain is not as wealthy as the United States and has "a unified parliamentary regime, a class structure far more rigid than that of the United States, and a spectrum of political ideologies far wider than America's" (Marmor and Klein 1986, 21). In the health care arena, the differences between Britain and the United States are apparent in the differing approaches to financing and controlling health care costs.

Fourth, and most important, the United Kingdom is eight years into a comprehensive health care reform program that entails some of the most sweeping changes to the venerable NHS since its creation half a century ago. The reform program is similar in some respects to that of the Netherlands in that it also draws its inspiration from Alain Enthoven's concepts of managed competition. In the context of the British health care system, such reform has involved infusing competition and consumer choice—or in Enthoven's terms, the creation of an internal market—into the NHS. Terms such as market and competition seem out of place in the NHS. It is this seeming contradiction that makes the NHS reform program so intriguing. The ways in which such similar competition-driven reforms play out in Britain and the Netherlands—two very different health care systems and societies—will clearly have important implications for comparative health care analysis.

The 1991 reform program, though the product of a conservative government, was quite radical in nature considering the environment into which it was introduced. Indeed, the UK government launched an ambitious reform program—of what was considered to be among the most static and impervious to change of all health care systems—based on what was essentially an untested theory.

The reforms could be viewed as "a design for health care delivery in the twenty-first century which would marry old-style British ideals of social justice with new-style American ideas about competition" (Day and

Klein 1989, 1) and move the British health care system into the uncharted territory of markets and competition in health care. As one British analyst pointed out prior to the implementation of the reform program, Britain is "lurching into a massive, uncontrolled experiment which will doubtless be fascinating for you all to monitor from the safe distance of this side of the Atlantic, if less exhilaratingly so for us who are going to live with it" (Culyer 1989).

The U.K. adoption of the "big bang" approach to health care reform (Klein 1995)—to boldly go where the NHS had never gone before, in one fell swoop, at a relatively rapid pace—sets the United Kingdom apart from other nations' incremental approach to health care reform (Chernichovsky 1995; Klein 1995). The impact of this conservative radicalism on the NHS and whether it creates "a new hybrid model of health care delivery" should be of interest to the United States (Charny et al. 1990).

The United Kingdom is located on the market-minimized pole of the health care continuum (Anderson 1989), since the central government plays a key role in health care planning and setting expenditure limits, and the majority of the population receives health care services from a wholly government-run and publicly financed entity. It would seem, however, that both poles of the continuum are turning in on each other, as Britain modeled the most significant restructuring in the history of the popular NHS on concepts such as competition that drive the U.S. health care system. In the United Kingdom market forces were introduced into a highly centralized, directly managed health care system that was already among the least expensive, most comprehensive, and equitable among the industrialized countries (Light 1997). Indeed, the evolution of what one analyst terms the "Americanization" of the NHS (Mechanic 1995) merits close attention by observers on both sides of the Atlantic.

OVERVIEW OF BRITISH HEALTH CARE

The British health care system stands out as the most centrally managed and financed health care system in the world—"an anomaly" among western industrialized nations (Anderson 1989, 42). This central management, finance, and budgeting can actually be described using the vocabulary of managed care, as health policy expert Donald Light did when he pointed out that the NHS

> can be regarded as one giant managed care system that had already accomplished most of the efficiencies now being achieved by American managed care systems through roughly similar means: tight, careful control over availability and distribution of specialty teams, service and facilities; a strong, broad foundation of primary care services that controlled access to specialty services and coordinated them; a mixture of capitation, salary and unit budgets for physicians . . . and tight budgets. (Light 1997, 301)

FIGURE 7-1   Health Expenditures, United States and United Kingdom, 1971–1997
(as percentage of GDP)

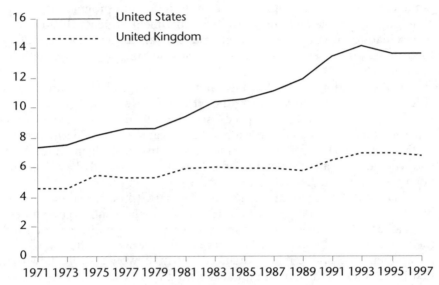

Source: OECD Health Data 98: A Comparative Analysis of 29 Countries. Paris: OECD/CREDES.

The NHS was once considered to be one of the best health systems in the world; it provides essentially cradle-to-grave care, regardless of one's ability to pay, and is free to the patient at the point of service. Yet long waiting lists, shortages of technology, decaying facilities, and underfunding have conspired to take off some of the lustre of the NHS. Despite its flaws, the NHS has retained popular support during its demicentury of existence.

The United Kingdom dedicates far less to health care than all other nations examined in this study; in 1997 it spent 6.7 percent of GDP on health care, one-half the amount that the United States spent that year (Figure 7–1) and one-third less on a per capita basis (Table 7–1). Despite spending half as much on health care as the United States, health status measures such as infant mortality and life expectancy reveal that the British and U.S. systems have similar outcomes. Given that the determinants of health status go beyond the financing levels of the health care system, however, it is important to note that such measures are limited in judging the overall performance of the health care system.

BRITAIN'S SACRED COW: THE NATIONAL HEALTH SERVICE

The NHS celebrated its fiftieth birthday in 1998, yet its origins go back even further. The 1911 National Health Insurance Act mandated limited

TABLE 7–1   Health Care in the United States and the United Kingdom

	United States	United Kingdom
Life expectancy at birth, 1995	72.7 (male)	74.4 (male)
	79.4 (female)	79.3 (female)
Median age of population, 1996	35	37
Projected percentage of population age 65 or older		
2000	12.5	15.9
2010	13.6	17.0
2020	17.5	19.7
Health care expenditures, 1997		
as % GDP	13.6	6.7
per capita	$4,090	$1,347
Distribution of health care spending, 1996 (as percentage of total spending)		
Hospitals	34	42 (1995)
Physicians	20	15.2 (1994)
Pharmaceuticals	8	17.5
Physicians per 1,000 persons, 1996	2.6	1.7 (1997)
Inpatient hospital beds per 1,000 persons, 1996	4.0	4.5
Average length of stay (days), 1996	7.8	9.8
Scanners per million persons, 1993	26.9	6.3
MRIs per million persons, 1995	16	3.4

Sources: OECD Health Data 98: A Comparative Analysis of 29 Countries. Paris: OECD/CREDES; World Bank.

medical coverage for low-income workers. But unlike the social insurance systems in Germany and Japan, the U.K. health insurance plan covered only general practitioners' services and excluded workers' dependents (Anderson 1989). From the 1920s through the 1940s, dissatisfaction with the insurance system grew, especially with respect to services provided during the war (Maynard 1990b).

The combination of postwar hardships and sense of solidarity in difficult times facilitated the creation of a comprehensive, national health service for the entire population (Anderson 1989). A report published in

1942 by the economist Lord Beveridge proposed reforming the social insurance system and laid out a blueprint for a "national health service. The health service was to be predicated on four principles: health services were to be (1) universal; (2) comprehensive; (3) free to the patient; and (4) financed by general tax revenues" (Anderson 1989, 28). The report reflected the environment of wartime shortages and rationing and demands for social welfare support from the government (Day and Klein 1989; Maynard 1990b). The enabling legislation to launch the NHS made its way through Parliament in 1946, with Minister of Health Aneurin Bevan arguing that "no society can legitimately call itself civilized if a sick person is denied medical aid because of a lack of means" (Lyall 1997b).

The legislation moved forward without the support of the British Medical Association; a poll taken that year revealed that more than half of all physicians surveyed opposed the NHS. Even two years later, just months before the official inauguration of the NHS, physician opposition was still very high (Rogaly 1989). To secure physician support for the nationalized health care system, Bevan got to the physicians through their wallets—"lined their teeth with gold," in his words. Physicians were offered the right to hold part-time hospital positions and have a private practice if they so chose. Bevan's assurance that physicians would not have to become salaried civil servants went far toward diffusing their opposition: Although some physicians left the country, the majority joined the new system (Anderson 1989).

The postwar Labour government had set in motion an extensive program of state ownership of major industries; nationalization of the health care system was one aspect of this strategy (Aaron and Schwartz 1984). Thus some 2,000 hospitals were nationalized (200 hospitals kept their private-sector status). There was a cost-control objective to this strategy, as it would allow the government to "gain some control over both the hospital-based specialists and the nonhospital-based general practitioners to limit the use of hospital services" (Potter and Porter 1989, 345).

The NHS, the world's first comprehensive national health care system, formally came into being in 1948. The NHS, the cornerstone of the British welfare state, was created in the nation that was at the forefront of the industrial revolution, a strong proponent of laissez-faire economics and an ardent supporter of limited government. The "planned economy for health" deviated from these positions (Anderson 1989).

NHS FINANCING

The chronic funding problems that have been the hallmark of the modern day NHS are actually an extension of the system's inability to keep up with demand from day one. NHS spending during its first year of existence was two-thirds more than planned, as Bevan remarked: "I shudder to think of the ceaseless cascade of medicine which is pouring down British throats at the present time" (*The Economist* 1998a). The establishment of a universal health service was predicated on the assumption that overall health costs would decline as easier access to a comprehensive range of services rendered the population healthier.

Even in the earliest days of the NHS there was a conflict between Bevan's vision of a free, comprehensive medical service and the pressure to introduce fees or charges for some services. For example, the Labour government legislated charges for prescription drugs in 1949 but never introduced them. Two years later, however, financial pressures led to the introduction of charges for dental services and glasses. Bevan resigned and Labor was defeated shortly thereafter (Smith 1998). The struggle to remain true to Bevan's ideal of a free comprehensive health service and the reality of the financing necessary to do so continues to this day.

The NHS is distinct from the private and social insurance programs discussed in earlier chapters in many facets, not least of all the financing aspect. Britain's NHS is financed almost completely from tax revenues, with only 2 percent of its budget coming from patient charges for eyeglasses, dental work, vision exams, and prescription drugs (Figure 7–2). Though there are copayments for prescription drugs, there are many exemptions for children, pregnant women, people aged 60 and older, and families on income support. Thus an estimated 80 percent of all prescriptions dispensed in 1998–1999 will be free. Patients pay 80 percent of the cost of dental treatment up to a ceiling of 340 pounds per course of treatment (Spencer and Associates 1998). Patient charges are also paid by nonnationals, by individuals purchasing private care in NHS facilities, and by individuals wishing to upgrade their accommodation in NHS facilities.

The two largest single-budget items are salaries for NHS staff and prescription drugs. The majority of NHS funds—approximately three quarters—are absorbed by the payroll of its million-strong workforce. Consider that an across-the-board raise of 3 percent increases the NHS wage bill by one billion pounds. After paying its workforce, the next largest single NHS expenditure item is drugs, which consume approximately one-tenth of the NHS budget (Hoare 1998; Murray 1998).[2]

---

[2] The U.K. government controls profits on pharmaceutical sales to the NHS through the pharmaceutical price regulation scheme, which covers all companies supplying drugs to the NHS. The scheme, which exempts new drugs, generic prescriptions, private prescriptions, and nonprescription medicines, regulates the amount of profit—measured as rate of return on capital—that drug companies can keep on their sales to NHS. Profits are kept within the range of 17 to 21 percent. The scheme also regulates price increases, the amount of advertising costs that can be passed through to the NHS, as well as the amount of R&D costs the companies can set against sales to the NHS (Earl-Slater 1997).

FIGURE 7-2   Sources of NHS Financing, 1996–1997 (in percentages)

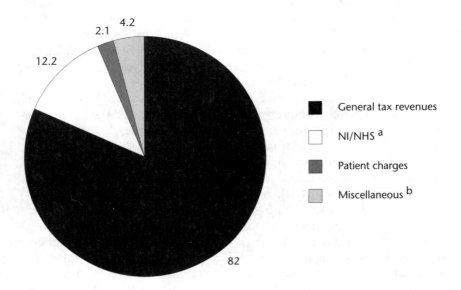

Source: Her Majesty's Stationary Office, Department of Health Report, "The Government's Expenditure Plans—1998–1999."

[a] NI/NHS refers to the National Insurance component of the Social Security payroll tax earmarked for the NHS.

[b] Miscellaneous includes repayments of principal on NHS Trust interest-bearing debt.

Tight budgetary control over finances is one of the better known features of the NHS. Though changes in how funds are allocated and controlled have been made, and more are being discussed, it is helpful to visualize NHS funds flowing into three separate pots. The lion's share of the funds (approximately 70 percent) goes into a budget allocated to eight regional health authorities and then further down to approximately 100 district health authorities (DHAs), each responsible for approximately 500,000 people. This cash-limited budget is determined according to a national capitation formula that takes into account each DHA's target population's demographics as well as various other factors. This budget funds hospitals and community health services, including hospital specialists. The second budget pot represents approximately one quarter of all NHS funds: a national GP contract covering all primary care services, including drugs, vision, and dental services. Finally, a separate pot of revenues covers community-based services, including nursing homes and home care for elderly patients (Jewell 1997; Light 1997).

The top-down budgetary process means that the "British government essentially decides how much health care the British people should consume every year" (Willets 1989, 66). The NHS's reputation for being parsimonious is evident in the fact that it provides comprehensive services to a population one-fifth the size of the U.S. population while spending one-fifteenth of what the United States spends (Light 1997).

Limits on health budgets have collided head-on with a growing demand for health services by the population. The U.K. health care system faces the same pressures as the U.S. system, including an aging population, the high cost of advanced technology, and the increased incidence of serious diseases such as AIDS and cancer. As in Canada, limits on the availability of medical technology and certain forms of treatment result in rationing by queue.

Waiting lists have been a persistent feature of the NHS since its inception; the NHS was created in an environment of postwar rationing of all goods and services. Yet as the wartime experience of shared hardship faded from memory, public willingness to wait for certain surgical procedures has steadily declined and the "democracy of the till [became] more attractive than the equity of the queue" (Day and Klein 1989, 27; Klein 1995; Willets 1989). As of the end of March 1998 nearly 1.5 million people were waiting for treatment for such procedures as hernia repair, varicose veins treatment, hip replacements, and cataract removal, up from 900,000 in the early 1990s. Though the waiting list has grown significantly, the average length of time a patient has to wait for treatment has held fairly steady since the 1960s at between thirteen and fourteen weeks (*The Economist* 1998b).

Perhaps the most frequently cited example of rationing in the NHS is that featured in Aaron and Schwartz's controversial 1984 study on the availability of various medical procedures, which compared U.S. and U.K. rates of hemodialysis (among other procedures). The study revealed that the overall rate of kidney dialysis treatment in Britain was approximately one-third that of other Western European countries and the United States. The age of the patient was seen to be a limiting factor, as British dialysis rates for patients under age 45 were equal to that of patients in the United States and Western Europe, but the rates declined as the patient's age increased. Kidney dialysis treatment for patients age 65, for example, was performed at a rate approximately one-tenth that of other nations (Aaron and Schwartz 1984). Although Britain does not have a formal, explicit age limit for dialysis treatment, it is clear that certain "policy decisions are implicitly made based on budget allocations" (Potter and Porter 1989, 351).

Critics have taken issue with Aaron and Schwartz, arguing that the study neglected the higher rate of home treatment and transplantation for kidney disease in Britain (Potter and Porter 1989). Moreover, critics contend that the underlying assumptions of the study—that the U.S. system is the baseline standard against which Britain should be measured—may be flawed because of evidence that overprovision of services may occur in the United States (Marmor and Klein 1986).

Finally, others have argued that the United States focuses on rationing in Britain while more than 40 million people lack health insurance in the United States, an example of rationing by ability to pay. It appears that rationing is in the eyes of the beholder: To the British, the necessity of insurance benefits to attain access to care in the United States would be considered rationing (Potter and Porter 1989).

Perhaps one of the more interesting aspects of the limits on availability of services in the NHS is how the politicians are shielded from blame: The medical profession essentially bears the brunt of rationing decisions. They have accepted this burden in exchange for a high degree of professional autonomy. Thus although it is the politicians' budgetary decisions that result in limits on resources, such political decisions emerge as clinical decisions by the physicians (Klein 1998, 122).

HEALTH CARE DELIVERY

General practitioners (GPs) are independent contractors working under a general contract negotiated between the British Medical Association and the Department of Health, and hospital specialists (consultants) are salaried employees of the hospital. As in Germany, there is a sharp separation between hospital physicians and GPs. As discussed further, the reforms enacted in the late 1980s to create an "internal market" within the NHS separated the purchase of health care services from the provision. To this end, certain large GP practices (known as GP fundholders) were given the option of having a fixed budget with which to buy specific services for their patients, and certain NHS hospitals became self-governing trusts, competing with other hospitals for contracts from health authorities and GP fundholders to provide services for patients.

PHYSICIANS AND HOSPITALS

There are 1.7 physicians per 1,000 population in the United Kingdom—the lowest physician-to-population ratio of all the nations in this study. General practitioners (GPs) form the backbone of the NHS, representing 60 percent of all physicians and handling 90 percent of all episodes of patient care (Maynard and Bloor 1996). All citizens and permanent residents are entitled to receive health services and are free to enroll with the GP of their choice. Although not everyone does, most people sign up with a GP, typically one located close to home. GPs are the patient's first point of contact with the system; they make the initial diagnosis and determine whether a patient will see a specialist, known in NHS parlance as a *consultant*. The majority of all prescription drug expenditures (80 percent) originate with GPs.

The average GP has nearly 2,000 patients in his or her practice (White 1995). Though publicly financed, GPs are independent self-employed entrepreneurs who work under terms of a contract that is negotiated nationally between the government and the medical profession through the British Medical Association. The entrepreneurial aspect is evident in the fact that more than 60 percent of the NHS 11,500 primary health care centers and clinics are owned by GPs (Hoare 1998).

GP compensation features a mix of capitation, salary, and fees. The capitation portion is derived by the number of patients on a physician's list and, prior to the reforms, represented nearly half of a physician's income. A second component covers the fixed costs of operating a practice. Finally, GPs receive fees for certain services such as maternity care, vaccinations, tests, and so forth (Maynard 1990b; Potter and Porter 1989).

As in Germany and Japan, there is a distinct separation between GPs and hospital physicians. Hospital consultants (specialists) have the choice of taking a full-time position with the NHS or a part-time position. If they choose the latter, there are no limits on the amount of time they can spend in private practice, providing they fulfill their "fixed" time commitments to the NHS.

In the prereform era these hospital specialists ruled the roost; in Donald Light's words, specialists in essence had "impenetrable fiefdoms" (Light 1997, 302). As salaried employees of the hospital, they were not necessarily responsive to GPs and their patients. The reforms have changed all that, shifting the balance of power away from specialists, as discussed later.

The NHS owns and operates more than 2,000 hospitals. As in Canada and elsewhere, the hospital sector has undergone significant contraction, with the number of inpatient beds falling from 8 per 1,000 population in 1982 to 4.5 in 1996 (OECD 1998).

Hospitals under the prereform NHS were run by District Health Authorities (DHAs). The reforms, as discussed further below, divorced the financing of health care from the provision, and the majority of hospitals became semi-independent entities, known as NHS Trusts.

In addition to the NHS hospitals, there are approximately 300 private hospitals, two-thirds of which are run by for-profit organizations and the remainder by charitable organizations. Less than 10 percent of all acute hospital beds in England are private beds, and these are devoted almost entirely to elective surgery. One quarter of the private beds are in public institutions—the private wards of NHS hospitals (OECD 1992).

FIGURE 7-3   Ownership of Residential Homes for Elderly Individuals, 1980 and
1994

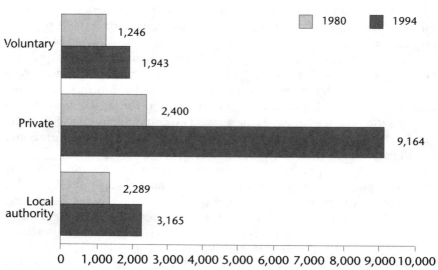

Source: Derek Terry and R. Starbridge, *Industry Sector Analysis: U.K. Health Care Service.* London: American Embassy, 1997.

LONG-TERM CARE SERVICES

Beginning in 1990, the government significantly curtailed its involvement in the long-term care arena. Local authorities currently apply a means test to determine whether individuals will pay for their own care or receive subsidized services.

Individuals with assets of fewer than 10,000 pounds, including the value of their home, have their care in a residential or nursing home paid for by the state through local authorities. Individuals with assets of up to 16,000 pounds must pay a share of the costs, and those with assets beyond that amount pay the full cost. Given that the annual tab for long-term care can easily reach 20,000 pounds per year, elderly individuals are often forced to sell their homes to cover the costs of care, a problem that also occurs in the United States (Spencer and Associates 1998).

The majority of institutionalized elderly patients are cared for either in public community homes or in private nursing homes (as opposed to geriatric wards of the NHS). Whereas in the acute sector, private providers represent a small portion of total health care services, they have virtually taken over the institutional long-stay elderly care sector (Figure 7–3). From 1980 to 1994, the number of private nursing homes more than quadrupled.

Long-term care in the United Kingdom, as elsewhere, is receiving increased attention because of the aging of the population. The government appointed a Royal Commission to look into long-term care financing. The commission's report, released in March 1999, recommended that nursing and personal care services for elderly individuals not in hospitals should be provide free of charge and financed by taxes. This proposal was in direct response to the situation in which many elderly people found themselves: having to sell their homes to pay for health care services (Timmons 1999).

THE ROLE OF THE PRIVATE SECTOR

The creation of the NHS did not entail the outlawing of private insurance for those benefits covered by the national plan, as the Canadian system did. And unlike Germany, where citizens can opt out of the public plan if their incomes are high enough, British citizens cannot opt out of the plan by not paying taxes (Anderson 1989). Thus they move between the NHS and the private sector. Indeed, the lines between public and private are fuzzy because a private patient may be treated in a private bed—known as a "pay bed"—in an NHS facility. And an individual patient may begin his or her course of treatment in the private sector and end up in the NHS if there are complications, the medical condition warrants treatment beyond the scope of services available in the private sector, or if a person's private medical insurance will not cover the treatment.[3]

Surveys indicate that the most common reason people take out private medical insurance is to avoid waiting for elective surgery. As Aaron and Schwartz pointed out, "The private patient pays to avoid waiting, the NHS patient waits to avoid paying" (Aaron and Schwartz 1984, 23). Private medical coverage is also a by-product of patients' desires for control over such specific aspects as the timing of an operation, the particular surgeon to perform the operation, and the particular hospital in which the procedure is performed (Day and Klein 1989).

Less than 5 percent of the population was covered by private insurance in 1979, and by 1984 private coverage rates had increased to just under 8 percent. The growth rate accelerated during the 1980s, and as of 1990, approximately 12 percent of the population was covered by private medical insurance. Between 1978 and 1988, the number of beds in private hospitals increased 50 percent (Day and Klein 1989). Though the share of the population with private medical insurance has held steady at between 12 and 13 percent, many individuals pay out-of-pocket for private treat-

---

[3] I am grateful to my colleague Chris Brown for clarification of this point.

ment and thus are not captured in these numbers. On the other hand, it is important to note that rates of private medical coverage vary significantly across Britain; in London, for example, private medical insurance rates approach 20 percent, but are as low as 5 percent in Scotland.[4]

The growth of private medical insurance coverage indicates that there are insufficient services within the NHS, causing patients to look elsewhere for care, yet it is important to remember that private sector care is specialized and limited to such elective (nonemergency) surgical procedures as hernias, varicose vein surgery, and hip replacements. Nearly 20 percent of all elective surgery is performed in the private sector (Marmor and Klein 1986; Pike 1989b).

Approximately 60 percent of private medical insurance coverage is provided by employers.[5] Employer-sponsored medical insurance is a taxable benefit to the employee; the employer-paid premium is treated as a tax-deductible business expense, and the employee pays taxes on the premium paid on his or her behalf (unless the employee earns less than 8,500 pounds per year).

In an effort to expand insurance coverage for elderly individuals, the government introduced tax relief in 1990 for private medical insurance for those age 60 and older. The Labour government, arguing that tax relief had not achieved its intended purpose, abolished it in 1997 (Curphy 1998; Eaglesham and Parker 1997).

Two large commercial insurers cover more than two-thirds of those covered by private medical insurance: PPP and Guardian Health recently merged and now cover 35 percent of the market, with British United Provident Association (BUPA) close behind with 34 percent of the market in 1997 (down from nearly 60 percent in 1985; U.S. Office of Fair Trading 1998).

BUPA's premiums rose dramatically in the 1980s; between 1980 and 1987 premiums rose 186 percent, and the retail price index rose 53 percent (Day and Klein 1989). Private insurers began to look to their American counterparts for cost-containment strategies. For example, BUPA entered into a strategic alliance with U.S. Healthcare and set up its own preferred provider network in 1996; PPP followed suit a year later.

NHS REFORMS: *WORKING FOR PATIENTS*

During the 1980s the cracks in the NHS system became increasingly evident: Concerns over declining quality, the closing of hospital wards be-

---

[4] I am grateful to my colleague Chris Brown for clarifying this point.

[5] A recent survey of nearly 900 companies revealed that one-third of responding companies provide private medical insurance for more than half of their work forces (Spencer and Associates 1998).

cause of lack of funds, long waiting lists for certain surgical procedures, nurses' strikes, and pervasive morale problems were just a few signs of an overloaded system (Day and Klein 1989). The number of patients on waiting lists continued to increase even as more funds were being pumped into the system.

Periodic attempts to restructure the NHS in the early 1980s were shelved. Indeed, there was always a significant risk attached to any effort to reshape the NHS, as the system was popular despite its obvious weaknesses, provided cradle-to-grave services, and thus touched the lives of every British citizen. It was assumed that "politicians tamper with the NHS at their peril" (Pike 1990d).

Former Prime Minister Margaret Thatcher was certainly never one to shy from controversy, however, and at her request a review of the NHS was conducted in 1988. Many NHS reform proposals were considered, focusing either on the creation of an insurance-based health care system to replace the tax-financed NHS or ways to make best use of the existing resources within the NHS through structural modifications (Day and Klein 1989).

The Thatcher government's review of the NHS culminated in a White Paper (precursor to legislation) published in January 1989, titled *Working for Patients*, which contained the broad strokes of significant NHS reforms (U.K. Department of Health 1989). The reforms drew heavily on U.S. economist Alain Enthoven's vision of an internal market that formed the centerpiece of his hallmark managed competition strategy. According to Enthoven's master plan, market forces would be introduced into the NHS, providers would be divided into separate groups, and the ensuing competition among them would increase the NHS's efficiency, thereby allowing the system to essentially provide more services for the same amount of money. Despite these significant changes, the funding basis of the NHS was left completely unchanged: The system was to remain tax-financed.

The White Paper set off a firestorm of protest, as doctors and other medical professionals, as well as the public, opposed the government's proposed reforms. Thatcher effectively ignored calls from the medical profession for increased funding to solve NHS problems, countering that lack of management and competition were the real source of the system's ills. Polls indicated that the public believed the controversial reforms would result in cuts in services, and heralded the end of public sector health care. Many believed the reforms represented the thin edge of the privatization wedge, and were merely a continuation of the selling spree of such state-run entities to the private sector as British Airways, British Steel, and Rolls Royce (Blendon and Donelan 1989). Indeed, the health reforms were seen as the third pillar of Thatcher's social revolution, which entailed education reforms, the poll tax, and NHS restructuring (Melcher and Maremont 1989; Rule 1990).

But Thatcher, turning a deaf ear to the opposition of the medical profession, the media, and the opposition parties, successfully imposed NHS
reforms by legislative fiat; President Bill Clinton could only have dreamed
of his health reform program speeding down the legislative track as swiftly
as Thatcher's did, propelled by her automatic majority in the legislature
and guided by her firm belief in the power of the market to cure the NHS
of its ills (Klein 1995).

The NHS reforms represented an unlikely combination of conservatism and radicalism (Day and Klein 1989), but did not change the four
original principles that created the NHS—that care be universal, comprehensive, free at the point of service, and financed by taxes. Indeed, even
Thatcher rejected the privatization option, and her proposals did not de-
part from the policy positions expressed during the 1980s calling for
tighter management control over the NHS. But at the same time, the proposals were quite radical because they aimed to reshape the NHS through
competition and patient choice—essentially infusing market principles
into a publicly financed health service that provides care in public institutions (Day and Klein 1989; Willets 1989, 65).

Another paradoxical feature of the health reforms is that they came
out of an environment of relative frugality in terms of health care expenditures, particularly compared to other nations such as the United States
and Canada. Although U.S. health care reform proposals were shaped in
large part by efforts to stem escalating health care expenditures, U.K. expenditures were among the lowest in the industrialized world and were
kept in check to a greater extent than in other nations. For example, during the period leading up to the reform program (1980–1987), when U.S.
health care expenditures as a percentage of GDP increased from 9.1 to
11.1 percent, U.K. expenditures remained fairly flat, increasing only from
5.3 to 5.9 percent of GDP.

The reforms aimed to make the best out of the consequences of tight
budgets; as Maynard explained, the reforms aimed to "minimize costs and
maximize benefits" within the NHS (Maynard 1995).

REFORMS AS EXPERIMENTAL SURGERY

The reforms detailed in the White Paper were enshrined in the 1990 National Health Service and Community Care Act and took effect in April
1991. The first step toward the creation of an internal market within the
NHS was to separate health care supply from demand, essentially creating
two distinct entities, one that would be responsible for the purchasing of
health care and the other for its provision.

This so-called purchaser–provider split was accomplished by radical
changes on both the demand and supply side of the health care equation.

On the demand side, purchasing would be the domain of groups of GPs with budgets. Known as fundholders, these GPs were allocated budgets with which to buy certain nonemergency services for their patients. In addition, newly recast DHAs would be responsible for contracting with providers to purchase services for their patients. Newly formulated "self-governing trusts" (former NHS hospitals), fundholding and nonfundholding GPs,[6] and private-sector providers filled out the supply side. The reforms further blurred the lines between public and private, because newly formed NHS trusts were encouraged to attract private patients in addition to NHS patients, and private hospitals were to compete for contracts from NHS purchasers to provide services to NHS patients (Ham 1996).

THE PURCHASERS

In the primary care sector, general practitioners with large practices (initially the limit was set at 11,000 patients, rather quickly reduced to 9,000, then whittled down to 7,000, and finally to 5,000) were given their own budgets, which would be set according to factors related to the composition of their patient list. GPs used these budgets to purchase a defined set of health care services for their patients, such as prescription drugs, diagnostic services, elective surgery, and outpatient care, operating in effect like small-scale HMOs. GP fundholders were to shop around for the best services for their patients that could be purchased from either public or private providers (Culyer 1989; Day and Klein 1989, 1991).

GP fundholders with a budget surplus at the end of the year could plow that money back into their practices (though not into their own pockets). That physicians could not personally benefit from any budget surplus served to counter concerns that the introduction of financial incentives would have an adverse impact on medical practice (Day and Klein 1991; Ham 1996). At the same time, GPs were protected from financial risk given that any expenditures in excess of 5,000 pounds per patient in any given year would be covered by the health authorities (Ham 1996).

The establishment of budget-holding GP practices represented a radical change for the NHS. The reforms encouraged GPs to compete for patients by increasing the share of income derived from capitation from less than 50 to 60 percent. The theory was that competition among GPs for patients would make them more efficient health care providers so they could attract more patients and thereby increase their capitation income. Moreover, because GPs were to coordinate all services for their patients, this would strengthen the linkages between the primary and secondary care sectors (Weiner and Ferriss 1990).

---

[6] GP fundholders actually play a dual purchaser–provider role, because they not only provide primary care services but purchase other services for their patients as well (Ham 1996).

GP fundholders thus wore a variety of caps. They were primary care givers, gatekeepers to specialists, and now managers of budgets and purchasers of care, which in essence required them also to be part actuary, part accountant, and part entrepreneur (Maxwell 1996). Because GPs were ill-equipped in terms of budget management expertise, they hired staff to manage their budgets; they received an annual allowance in addition to their budgets to cover such managerial expenses (Ham 1996).

Fundholding took hold relatively quickly: By 1993 approximately one quarter of the population were members of a fundholding GP practice, and this share increased to one-third by the end of 1994. Indeed, GP fundholding—never considered to be the centerpiece of the reforms but rather the reform's "wild card"—actually turned out to be one of the reform program's shining stars (Robinson and LeGrand 1995). By 1997 more than half of all GPs were fundholders in more than 3,000 GP fundholding practices that covered one-half of the population—though it is important to note that the prevalence of GP fundholding varies significantly from region to region.

Though the overall impact of GP fundholding is difficult to assess and the evidence to date gives mixed messages, in general studies indicate that GP fundholders have been successful in reducing the amount of time their patients wait for outpatient hospital treatment; in increasing the efficiency of diagnostic services; and in reducing prescription expenditures (Ham 1996).

In terms of internal NHS power politics, GP fundholding has raised GPs from their underdog status with regard to hospital consultants. With fundholders holding the purse strings, consultants have been forced to become more accountable and responsive to GPs, who can opt to take their business elsewhere if the treatment is deemed unacceptable.

The reforms turned the DHAs into purchasers as well. In their former lives, DHAs organized and delivered care by running hospitals. Their new role recast them as purchasing agents for the patients in their area; approximately 100 health authorities are each responsible on average for a population of 500,000 people. Health authorities are allocated a budget based on a weighted capitation formula that they draw on to purchase all services for their patients *except* those covered by GP fundholders in their area. Whereas previously health authorities contracted only with the hospitals they directly managed, the new reform regime enabled health authorities to negotiate contracts with either NHS hospitals, private sector hospitals, or newly formed NHS self-governing trusts, depending on which offers the best price and quality of health care services. Health authorities also oversee the nonfundholding GPs in their area (Day and Klein 1989; Ham 1996; Prowse 1989a, 1990a).

Together with the GP fundholders, DHAs are in essence proxy consumers (Klein 1995) buying services on behalf of their populations. The difference between the two is that DHAs purchase most services for their populations, whereas GP fundholders purchase nonemergency care for patients.

THE PROVIDERS

The most significant change on the supply side of the health care reform equation was the ability of NHS hospitals to become what are known as NHS self-governing trusts. These trusts are independent of the DHAs to which all NHS hospitals previously reported. Though not privatized—they remained part of the NHS—they have much more freedom over their operations. For example, self-governing trusts are allowed to raise their own capital and have significant control over their own finances. Moreover, they employ their own staffs and thus can set pay levels and contract terms, liberating them from the highly centralized pay agreements that had been fixed on a national basis (Day and Klein 1989; Willman 1992).

The self-governing trusts are public organizations accountable to the Secretary of State for Health. No longer directly funded by the central government, trusts generate revenue by contracting with DHAs, other self-governing hospitals, as well as private insurers to provide their services. Trusts are expected to achieve a 6 percent return on assets (Maynard and Bloor 1996; Smee 1995).

Within the first year, 156 hospitals had become self-governing Trusts. By the end of 1994 there were more than 400 trusts responsible for 95 percent of all hospital and community health expenditures (OECD 1995; Smee 1995; Willman 1992). In addition to the NHS Trusts, private hospitals compete for private pay patients as well as for contracts for NHS patients.

MISSION IMPOSSIBLE?

The creation of an internal market within the centrally run NHS was more than a formidable challenge—it bordered on the impossible (Maynard 1993). Those involved in the health care sector clearly had little experience with competition and free-market principles. And even though the NHS had detailed budgets for health services, a serious dearth of information regarding the cost of services has stymied the creation of a competitive market in health care, which requires highly sophisticated data systems to not only determine appropriate prices but to evaluate and monitor health contracts and services. The transformation of the "primitive" information system of the NHS into a modern database responsive to the complex demands of a new competitive system has proven to be a daunting and expensive endeavor. Moreover, the purchasers are inexperienced in the role of educated buyers of health care services (Charny et al. 1990; Day and Klein 1991, 50; The Economist 1990; Light 1991a, 1997).

Not unexpectedly, the reforms actually necessitated increased expenditure levels to cover investments in qualified staff and new management information and billing systems. The number of managers in the NHS, for example, more than quadrupled between 1985 and 1991 (*The Economist* 1993; Prowse 1989a, 1989b, 1990a). Over the period 1989–1992 U.K. health care expenditures rose nearly 20 percent, from 5.8 percent of GDP to 6.9 percent. The NHS budgets for 1991–1992 and 1992–1993 featured the largest increases in more than ten years (Klein 1995; OECD 1998; White 1995).

TOWARD THE NHS'S NEXT HALF CENTURY

By the mid-1990s, with John Major at the helm rather than Margaret Thatcher, the lexicon of the reform program changed, revealing a shift in emphasis away from an ironclad dedication to the magic of the competitive market to a focus on cooperation between purchasers and providers. Purchasing was no longer referred to as such; rather, it became known as "commissioning" (Ham 1996).

The Labour Party ran its 1997 campaign on a platform of "Saving the NHS," promising to abolish the internal market, which they argued had spawned the twin evils of excessive bureaucracy and the associated administrative costs and the inequity resulting from fundholding patients getting preferential treatment over nonfundholding patients (Dixon and Mays 1997). In December 1997 newly elected Labour released its health reform manifesto titled, "The New NHS," which laid out a ten-year reform program. Despite Blair's pledge to abolish the internal market, one of the principal features of the internal market—the purchaser–provider split—will remain.

Labour's incremental approach is welcomed by many of the victims of "reform fatigue," brought on by nearly a decade of tumultuous change (Ham 1998a).

The changes Labour proposes will actually build on the success of GP fundholders, expanding fundholding to all GPs (though as one analyst pointed out, depending on your perspective, GP fundholding with be either "eliminated or universalized"; Klein 1998). GP fundholders will be replaced by 500 groups of GPs known as Primary Care Groups (PCGs). Each PCG will actually be made up of teams of GPs (up to fifty GPs) and community nurses responsible for approximately 100,000 people. Thus rather than covering one doctor or one practice's patients, these larger physician and nurse groups will be responsible for the entire population of a specific geographic region. Whereas GP fundholding was voluntary, participation in a PCG will be mandatory.

Given the costs involved in the annual contracting cycle, PCGs will have longer term contracts with providers of at three years in duration. PCGs will essentially take control of the NHS budget as of April 1999, providing all GP services as well as buying hospital and community care for their patients, including emergency treatment. The government expects that the lengthening of contracts combined with the consolidation of purchasers from more than 3,000 GP fundholders and 100 health authorities to the 500 PCGs will cut administrative costs.

For the first time in the history of the NHS, all health monies will be in a single sterling pot, tightly capped. Thus the PCGs will become in essence managed care organizations. This change further elevates the role of GPs within the NHS, for even though health authorities will have a critical role in determining where and what services are provided, GPs will be "in the driver's seat" (Dixon and Mays 1997; Klein 1998, 114; Timmons 1998).

If the key words of the Thatcher reforms were *choice* and *competition,* the key words for Blair's "new NHS" are *collaboration* and *cooperation.* Labour's preelection rhetoric focused on the need for reforms to tone down the harsher elements of the free market in the NHS and replace it with a kinder, gentler partnership. In reality, there was never much competition in the NHS. As Klein pointed out, because the NHS is tax financed, with the Minister of Health accountable to Parliament, "Decisions cannot be left to the market since ministers will be left with the consequences" (Klein 1998, 117). The government was continually monitoring the market and intervened frequently to mitigate against any adverse consequences of competition through regulatory measures in areas such as provider mergers, purchaser mergers, arrangements for handling providers in difficulty, and collusion (Ham 1996). In essence, the government kept the market on a short leash.

Moreover, as noted previously, a serious dearth of information and very shallow pool of expertise among NHS managers in competitive market principles did not advance the market's cause either. Finally, in contrast to the U.S. health care system, for example, where competition was able to feed off of the fat in the system, such an environment of excess capacity does not exist in the lean NHS. As Klein pointed out, "Importation of U.S. notions of competition in Britain meant transplanting ideas born in an environment of plenty into environment of scarcity" (Klein 1998, 117).

Labour's plans for the NHS's second half-century focus on keeping certain elements of the competitive reform program such as the purchaser–provider split, while at the same time reformulating the role of GP fundholders. As such they represent a compromise between the old command-and-control NHS and a Thatcherite ideal of a free market NHS (Dixon and Mays 1997; Parston and McMahan 1998).

FIGURE 7-4   Public and Private Share of Total Health Expenditures, Selected
              Countries, 1997

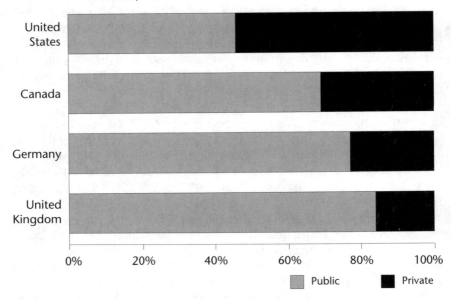

Source: OECD Health Data 98: A Comparative Analysis of 29 Countries. Paris: OECD/CREDES.

Neither the current nor past reforms address what many argue is the fundamental problem of the NHS: the constant struggle between budgetary limits and increasing patient demands. Indeed the core issue is understanding why the U.K. dedicates far fewer resources to health care than other industrialized nations (Day and Klein 1989; Light 1991a).

Brookings Institution economist Henry Aaron pointed out at the time when the initial NHS reform program was under consideration that "the idea that savings from competition are going to bail them out of the dilemma is nonsense. The British have to decide whether or not they are going to spend more of their wealth on modern health care" (cited in Lohr 1988). Ten years later Aaron's comment is still on the mark. The United Kingdom is unusual in its limited reliance on private funding—the lowest share of any of the other nations in this study (Figure 7–4). In the fall of 1997 the British Medical Association floated the idea of having patients pay 10 pounds per office visit. The resulting public outcry led to a government pledge to infuse more money into the NHS. But many see the increasing use of patient copayments as the only way out of the underfunding quagmire. John Willman argued in his recent book *A Better State of Health* that charges should be introduced for physician office visits, daily charges for hospital stays, with an extra charge for single rooms, and that significant reductions should be made in the number of exemptions for prescription drug copayments. Indeed, if the government chooses not to raise taxes to provide increased revenue, the NHS may be forced to turn to private sector funds (Murray 1998b; D. Smith 1998).

CONVERGENCE

The reforms of the past decade have thrown the NHS into a gray area, so that the system can no longer be simply typecast as a public system nor is it a private system. Thus it is moving closer to the health systems of every other nation in this study, which also evade such tidy classification. The blurring of the lines between public and private, the movement—to a certain degree—away from the centralized command-and-control system to one that shifts power further down to the local level, as well as the introduction of some elements of market-based systems, leads one to describe the NHS as a "politically managed health care market" (Ham 1996). It joins the Netherlands in its introduction of market principles under the keen eye of the government and even systems such as Germany's and Canada's where competition is being introduced within predominately publicly financed national health insurance systems.

Indeed, the NHS reforms can be viewed as part of a broader trend toward relying on management principles and practices to achieve greater health care efficiency and effectiveness (Day and Klein 1989). First the GP fundholders, and now the PCGs, move the U.K. system closer to certain American managed care practices. Yet as noted at the outset of this chapter, elements of U.S. managed care already existed in the NHS. Indeed, the NHS has what U.S. employer health purchasing coalitions seek: large purchasers for a given population "with a mandate to develop integrated strategies to meet the health needs of their population" (Light 1998).

Elements of U.S. managed care are evident in the private health care sector as U.K. private medical insurers have developed preferred provider organizations similar to U.S. arrangements. And recently the U.K. drew on American expertise in the development of telephone triage centers with the launch of 24-hour helplines within the NHS. The after-hours service, called NHS Direct, is staffed by nurses (Lazarus 1998).

Signs of convergence notwithstanding, fundamental differences will remain. In the final analysis, it would appear that cultural distinctions play a significant role in explaining differences between health care systems. Klein articulated the differences between the U.S. and U.K. health care systems:

> I have often argued that Britain is an "original sin" society, where we don't believe that the world can be totally put to rights. We accept problems and

are rather fatalistic about our capacity to deal with some of them. In contrast, America is a "perfectibility of man" society, where the view is that if there is a problem, you can solve it. (quoted in Potter and Porter 1989, 364)

Such cultural differences between the two societies—such as one's stronger confidence in its problem-solving abilities—are reflected in their approaches to health care and explain British patients' tolerance of waiting lists, as well as American insistence on trying every available medical procedure when someone is ill. These profound differences render any debate over the possibility of exporting the U.S. managed care system to Britain an exercise in futility "because it would mean trying to transplant cultural institutions between societies with totally different patterns of cultural values" (Rudolf Klein, quoted in Potter and Porter 1989, 364). Although it is clear that the United States and Britain have two very different systems that reflect their different cultures, a shared reliance on management principles within the health care sector transcends these differences. This is reflected in the prominence of managed care arrangements in the U.S. system and the evolving reform program within the NHS (Day and Klein 1989; Pike 1990a).

CHAPTER 8

International Experience and U.S. Health Care

This journey across the continuum of international health systems has revealed a broad range of approaches to the financing, organization, and delivery of health care. At the same time it has highlighted the challenges nations share in terms of how to tackle the universal conundrum of providing high quality care to their populations at a reasonable overall cost.

This study has also shown the 1990s was a decade of health care reform, and that the various reform measures adopted all share a common propellent: control over escalating health care costs—the "fiscal imperative," as health policy expert David Wilsford has called it. The need to control health care costs has driven change within all systems examined, fueling the widespread shift from traditional indemnity fee-for-service insurance into managed care plans in the U.S. health care system, the tightening of supply-side cost control mechanisms such as expenditure caps in Germany and Canada, and demand-side measures such as increased patient copayments in Japan. Certain market-based mechanisms have been introduced to varying degrees in systems that previously accorded no role to the market in health care.

The blend of free-market competition and government regulation in the form of managed markets or regulated competition in the health care sector has emerged as a popular course of treatment in many nations. The major reform programs undertaken in nations such as the United Kingdom and the Netherlands have not, however, significantly changed the predominantly public financing arrangements that underpin their health care systems, nor have such changes affected universal access. Although the invisible hand of the market has more maneuverability than before, it is still kept in check to a far greater degree by the gloved hand of government regulation than is the case in the U.S. system. It remains to be seen whether this "marriage of medical markets and social welfare universalism" (Morone and Goggin 1995, 568) will be one of wedded bliss or marital strife.

Although the systems studied have adopted different approaches to confronting shared challenges, it is clear that no ideal health system ex-

TABLE 8–1   Total Health Expenditures and Health Outcome Measures

	Total health expenditures % GDP	Life expectancy at birth		Infant mortality
		Males	Females	
United States	13.6	72.7	79.4	7.8
Germany	10.4	73.6	79.9	5
Canada	9.3	75.4	81.5	6
Netherlands	8.5	74.7	80.4	5.2
Japan	7.3	77.0	83.6	3.8
United Kingdom	6.7	74.4	79.3	6.1

Source: OECD Health Data 98: A Comparative Analysis of 29 Countries. Paris: OECD/CREDES.

ists; each system has its shortcomings. Waiting lists within the U.K.'s NHS and Canada's provincial health care system, overprescription in Japan, and the more than 40 million people without health insurance coverage in the United States are but some of the more obvious blemishes on health care systems across the spectrum.

The United States spends more money on health care than any other nation, but does not fare any better in terms of health outcome measures such as life expectancy or infant mortality. Based on these measures, both of which are, at best, proxy indicators of the quality of health care being delivered to the populations of various nations, the level of health care expenditures and health outcomes would not appear to be strongly related (Table 8–1).

Some analysts argue that comparisons of infant mortality and life expectancy rates do not adequately reflect the quality of U.S. health care, however. These analysts point out that the American population is more heterogeneous than those of other countries, and poverty rates among children in the United States are higher than in Japan or Western Europe. They also note that Americans' drug, drinking, and smoking habits, as well as other lifestyle characteristics, may contribute to higher U.S. infant mortality and lower life expectancy figures.

Such demographic and lifestyle factors certainly must be taken into consideration. That the U.S. population differs markedly from those of the other nations examined in this study is undeniable. But these differences should not be used to dismiss the importance of understanding how other nations finance and organize their health care systems—and how that might affect health outcomes.

Examining the methods of health care organization and finance of other nations can also help "guard against ethnocentrism in explanation by identifying similarities in different systems" (Klein 1991, 283). All the health care systems analyzed in this study certainly face the shared problems of escalating health care costs, aging populations, and finite health resources. And although each system is and will remain unique, this study has revealed that some nations have also adopted similar approaches for addressing shared problems.

THE UNITED STATES IS UNIQUE

The continuum of health care systems stretches from the tightly budgeted, centrally run British National Health Service to the predominantly private, voluntary system in the United States, and includes the provincial government-administered Canadian national health insurance system and the public–private mix of government-mandated health insurance systems in Germany, Japan, and the Netherlands. The United States emerges as one of a kind because of a number of characteristics particular to American health care.

NATURE OF INSURANCE COVERAGE

Health care coverage in the United States is neither universal nor comprehensive. More than 43 million Americans lack health insurance coverage, and many millions more do not have adequate coverage against the high costs of health care. Nations that provide universal coverage to their populations have accomplished this through a combination of *compulsion and subsidization;* individuals are required to have health insurance, insurers are required to cover everyone, and cross-subsidization across risk groups allows the entire population to have health insurance coverage (Fuchs 1991).

The United States has not yet reached this point because it does not accept compulsion and subsidization—the two basic premises of social insurance. Ideological factors come into play, as national health insurance is denounced by many Americans as a form of socialism—although national health insurance was introduced in Germany and Japan as an *antidote* to the spread of socialism (Ikegami 1991; Starr 1992). As long as the United States withholds support for compulsion and subsidization—and the failure of the Clinton health reform proposal demonstrated the limited appeal of these concepts to most Americans—universal coverage will remain unattainable.

ROLE OF GOVERNMENT

The government is a much more active participant in the health care systems in nations other than the United States. Governments are directly involved in financing health care, as well as setting overall funding levels and establishing uniform fee schedules for physicians and annual budgets for hospitals. Although one expects this to be the case in the systems of the United Kingdom and Canada, it is also true in the predominantly private delivery systems of Germany, the Netherlands, and Japan. The government serves an important role in guaranteeing universal coverage, establishing uniform benefit levels, as well as exerting a powerful influence on cost-control processes. As health analyst Brian Abel-Smith pointed out, "It is acceptable for government to do the regulating . . . [and] there is no question of the regulated taking over the regulators" (Abel-Smith 1992, 415).

Though the German system, for example, relies heavily on negotiation, consensus, and self-regulation among the major health care groups, the threat—or what Uwe Reinhardt has called the "Damocles sword"—of stronger government intervention is always present (Reinhardt 1994). This threat became a reality with the 1993 reforms as the government lost faith, or patience, with the process of self-regulation and moved from the sidelines to actively tighten the reins of cost control.

Increased governmental involvement, however, went hand in hand with the movement to introduce such private-sector measures as competition among the sickness funds. Such competition is regulated in the sense that the risk equalization fund ensures that insurance funds compete for members on factors other than risk status. Indeed, it can be argued that the German government uses market mechanisms to achieve its cost-control goals: Patient cost sharing and competition among health funds are "policy tools at the disposal" of the government (Morone and Goggin 1995, 560).

The powerful interest groups supporting the trillion-dollar U.S. health care system, the diffusion of power among different U.S. governmental bodies and among different levels of government, and Americans' inherent mistrust of an expanded governmental role in health care as evidenced by the failure of the proposed Clinton health reform plan are all factors likely to preclude a significantly broader governmental role in the U.S. health care system.

HEALTH CARE FINANCING

All the other health care systems considered in this study rely on public financing to a greater extent than does the U.S. system. General tax revenues provide the bulk of health care financing in the United Kingdom and Canadian systems, and mandatory health insurance contributions or premiums based on income, and not risk status, finance the mixed systems of Germany, the Netherlands and Japan. Though the share of U.S. health expenditures covered by public financing has increased from 42 percent in 1990 to 46 percent today, it is still below the average of nearly 75 percent in the other nations analyzed in this book.

LIMITED CONVERGENCE AMONG SYSTEMS

We have seen that no perfect system exists nor does one pure system exist: No health care system is either a completely free-market, competitive system or a wholly regulatory system; rather, a combination of both features exists in all of the systems examined. The United States, whose system is closest to the free-market pole of the continuum, has debated (though to date not implemented) consumer-protection measures that would significantly increase governmental regulation at the federal level to address such perceived weaknesses of managed care arrangements such as limits on coverage and access to emergency care and specialists, to name just a few. The country at the market-minimized pole, the United Kingdom, has introduced significant market-based reforms into its health care system; the Netherlands has undertaken a health care reform program to introduce competition and patient choice into a system that was previously heavily regulated. These two countries have shaped their health care reforms based to varying degrees on the concept of managed competition, which also served as the basis of the failed Clinton health care reform proposals in the United States.

Though we see some signs of convergence among health care systems, it in some ways consists largely of a one-way convergence of other nations' systems toward that of the United States. It is important to emphasize that this is a *convergence of strategies* such as managed competition or regulated markets that shapes specific health care institutions rather than convergence among the health care institutions themselves (Klein 1991, 289). For example, even though the Netherlands and the United Kingdom have undertaken fairly radical health care reform programs, they have kept intact their nations' health care financing and delivery systems, backing away neither from universal coverage nor predominantly public income-based financing arrangements.

One way of looking at the reform process across the spectrum is to consider what policy analyst David Wilsford has referred to as a "convergence of philosophy and goals" coupled with a "divergence of organizational principles and instruments" (Wilsford 1995, 578). All of the nations in this study, except the United States, share the view of health care as a public good, and thus ensure universal access and accord the government a larger role within the health care system—even though the organizations and institutions used to achieve these goals differ from nation to nation. The United States, in contrast, has a rather unique ability to apparently tolerate a significant share of its population going without health insurance coverage and in the process facing considerable obstacles to receiving necessary health care services. On the other hand, all of the nations in this study, including the United States, are considering similar strategies for controlling costs and achieving other desirable health outcomes.

Managed care, contrary to popular perception, is not an American invention. Arrangements similar to HMOs covered large segments of the population throughout Europe at the beginning of the century. We saw, for example, that closed panels were common until being banned in Germany. As health policy expert Abel-Smith pointed out, "President Nixon reinvented a very old wheel" (Abel-Smith 1988, 715). Certain features of managed care, such as capitation as a method of physician payment as well as the use of general practitioners as gatekeepers, are evident in many of the systems studied.

Though nations such as Germany and the Netherlands are experimenting with other features of U.S.-style managed care such as selective-contracting, disease management, pharmacy benefit management, and so on, other nations are unlikely to embrace managed care as fully as has the United States; rather, they will pick and choose from managed care's tool box and apply specific procedures to improve quality, enhance efficiency, or control costs within the confines of their universal, publicly financed systems.

AGING POPULATIONS

One area in which there is undeniable convergence is in the shifting demographic makeup of the nations examined. The aging of the population raises a host of issues from long-term care to increases in the use of pharmaceuticals and high-technology medicine. Health care spending increases markedly after age 45; consider that health care spending on men aged 45 to 54 is nearly 50 percent higher than for men aged 35 to 44, and men aged 55 to 64 spend twice as much as men aged 35 to 44.

The top trend lines in Figure 8–1 shows which of the nations examined have set up long-term care programs for their populations. Japan and Germany share particularly troubling demographic straits. The fertility rate in both Japan and Germany is significantly below the "replacement rate" needed to maintain a constant population. Population aging and negative population growth will have a chilling effect on health programs funded on a pay-as-you-go basis.

Population aging will also have an impact on prescription drug and medical technology use. Japan is already a heavy consumer of prescription drugs, reflecting among other things a cultural preference for pharmaceu-

FIGURE 8-1   Actual and Projected Percentage of the Population Aged 65 and Older, Selected Countries, 1990–2030

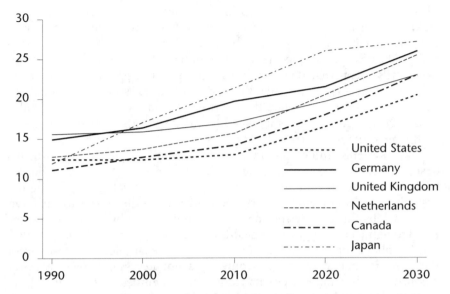

Source: United Nations, Population Division, *Sex and Age Quinquennial 1950–2050* (1998 edition).

tical interventions over surgery. We also saw that physicians play a dual role as pharmacist, dispensing nearly three quarters of all the drugs they prescribe, and deriving more than half of their incomes from doing so. Most of the nations examined have implemented measures to control rising drug costs; for example, in Germany the reference price system is coupled with specific expenditure caps on prescription drugs that physicians exceed at their own financial peril. German drug expenditures, which increased at an average annual rate of 10 percent in the 1980s, have slowed to 1 percent. In Japan, mandatory price cuts took effect in April 1998, reducing the cost of more than 1,500 drugs by an average of nearly 10 percent; drug expenditures declined 4 percent from 1997 to 1998. Further price cuts are expected with the introduction of a reference price system forecast for 2000 (Luesby 1998). In contrast, drug sales in the United States have risen nearly 17 percent this year, more than four times the increase in overall health care expenditures. Although the Untied States does not face a population aging crisis as imminent as Germany's or Japan's, demographic pressures clearly will force the United States as well to wrestle more seriously with the issues of long-term care and prescription drug costs in the relatively near future.

THE FUTURE OF U.S. HEALTH CARE

This survey of the complex workings of international health systems yields several important lessons for the United States. The experience of the various nations surveyed with universal, comprehensive health insurance indicates that the existence of national health insurance does not necessarily mean that the government controls the practice of medicine, nor does it necessarily involve limits on the patient's choice of provider. International experience should also correct the misconception that health insurance systems that are mandated by the government must also be run by the government.

The systems studied provide working examples of health care systems designed and financed according to the simple rule that all individuals must contribute according to ability to pay. The central tenet guiding the systems and guaranteeing universal access is that of the cross-subsidization of the sick by the healthy and the lower income by the higher income earners. Though a separate private health insurance track is available to those earning above the income limit in Germany, for example, the one-tenth of the population that takes that route does not necessarily receive better medical care but rather benefits from more amenities and a higher level of comfort (Reinhardt 1994; White 1995). Thus these systems provide evidence of the range of what is possible, as discussed at the beginning of this book.

Perhaps one of the most important lessons provided by international experience detailed is that health care reform is an ongoing, dynamic process. Germany, for example, has been fighting the health care cost-control battle for more than twenty years, during which time the government has passed more than a dozen major health reform measures. Its health care system is a centenarian, yet Germany continues to introduce new changes to refine the system and sharpen its cost-control tools, all the while preserving universal access to comprehensive health care benefits. In the Netherlands, the decade that has passed since the Dekker reform proposals were first introduced has been marked by constant tinkering and forward and backward steps.

The United States turned away from a dramatic change in its health care system, including a broader role for government, with the speedy rejection of the Clinton reform plan. More than five years later, concerns have increased about whether the subsequent widespread transformation from traditional fee-for-service delivery methods to a wide array of managed care arrangements (Figure 8–2) necessitate some degree of increased governmental regulation. The brave world of managed care-dominated health plans dodged the legislative bullet this year, but legislative mea-

FIGURE 8-2   Percentage of Uninsured Americans Covered by Managed Versus Unmanaged Care, 1988–1998

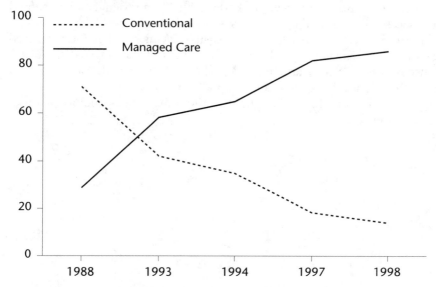

Sources: "Health Benefits in 1998." *KPMG* (June 1998).

sures falling under the broad rubric of patients' rights are likely to be enacted in the next Congress.

Whereas managed care is certainly not without its shortcomings, it is but one part of the larger health care system. Reform efforts need to target the shortcomings of managed care as well as the shortcomings of the system as a whole—notably the lack of universal coverage.

Ultimately the problems associated with managed care as the predominant mode of health care delivery and financing must be considered separately from the access problem. Managed care has done what it set out to do—help employers get a handle on escalating health care costs. It was developed as a cost-control strategy aimed at those already covered—not as a means to cover the uninsured (Buchanan 1998).

The access problem is the most serious systemic problem requiring governmental attention. Despite the enactment of incremental measures aimed at making insurance coverage more portable and targeting certain populations such as uninsured children, the ranks of the uninsured have swelled at the rate of one million per year over the past several years. In the current environment of relatively strong economic growth coupled with low unemployment, the question is, "If not now, when?"

The United States, unlike the other nations in this study, has a marked ambivalence about whether health care is a right to which all Americans are entitled. Thus in a variation of "don't kill the messenger," one should not necessarily blame the delivery system—managed care—for the failure of the U.S. society to reach the consensus that most other industrialized nations have managed to achieve. Uwe Reinhardt has referred to such a consensus as a "clearly articulated social ethic" that health care is a social good that should be made available to all (Reinhardt 1997). Any systemic reform process to address the plight of the uninsured is doomed without such consensus.

APPENDIX   Six Systems at a Glance

	United States	Germany	Japan	Netherlands	Canada	United Kingdom
Total health expenditure as % GDP						
1980	9.1	8.8	6.4	7.9	7.3	5.6
1990	12.6	8.7	6.0	8.3	9.2	6.0
1997	13.6	10.4	7.3	8.5	9.0	6.7
Total health expenditure per capita[1]						
1980	$1,086	$ 649	$ 524	$ 679	$ 717	$ 444
1990	$2,799	$1,279	$1,082	$1,326	$1,696	$ 955
1997	$4,090	$2,339	$1,741	$1,825	$2,095	$1,347
Life expectancy at birth (years)						
Females	79.4	79.9	83.6	80.4	81.5	79.3
Males	72.7	73.6	77.0	74.7	75.4	74.4
At age 65 (years)						
Females	18.9	18.6	21.5	18.6	20.2	18.4
Males	15.7	14.9	16.9	14.4	16.3	14.7
Infant mortality[2]	7.8	5.0	3.8	5.2	6.0	6.1

APPENDIX *(Continued)*

	United States	Germany	Japan	Netherlands	Canada	United Kingdom
Aging demographics Projected percent of the population aged 65+						
2000	12.5	16.2	16.5	14.1	12.3	15.9
2020	17.5	22.5	25.6	21.5	18.2	19.7
Median age of the population	35	37.6	40	36	35	37
Coverage Percent of the population with health insurance coverage	61.4% employer-sponsored plans; 8.7% other private coverage; 13.2% Medicare; 10.8% Medicaid; 3.2% military; 16.1% uninsured	91% of the population covered by mandatory social insurance[3]; 9% have private insurance	100% of the population covered by mandatory public social insurance (65% employment related plans; 35% plans for self-employed, unemployed, retirees)	63% of the population covered by mandatory social insurance; 5% civil servants insurance; 32% private insurance; 100% population covered under national catastrophic care program	100% of the population covered under provincial health insurance plans; the majority of the population has supplemental insurance coverage	100% of the population covered through National Health Service; approximately 10% of the population has private supplemental insurance coverage
Health care financing Percent that is						
Public	46	78	78	72	69	84
Private	54	22	22	28	31	16

Role of the employer/income-based premiums for social insurance (as percentage of salary)	Mandatory hospital insurance (HI) payroll tax finances part A of the Medicare program: 1.45 employer 1.45 employee[4]	Contribution rate varies by sickness fund; 1997 average was: 6.75 er 6.75 ee	Contribution rate varies by insurance fund; 1997 average was: 4.2 er 4.2 ee	Contribution rate set by the government; 1999 rate was: 5.85 % er 1.55 % ee plus 10.25 % ee for long-term catastrophic care program	General federal and provincial tax revenues. Majority of employers sponsor supplemental medical insurance programs for their employees.	General tax revenues. Employers sponsor supplemental medical insurance programs, typically for executives and their dependents.
As % of total health expenditures:[5]						
Hospitals	34 (a)	35 (b)	29 (c)	53 (a)	34 (a)	42 (c)
Physicians	20 (a)	16 (b)	34 (c)	9 (b)	14 (a)	15 (d)
Pharmaceuticals	8 (a)	13 (b)	20 (a)	11 (a)	14 (a)	17 (a)
Physicians						
Physicians per 1,000 population	2.6 (b)	3.4 (b)	1.8 (b)	2.6 (g)	1.8 (a)	1.7 (a)
Physician consultations per capita	6.0 (b)	6.4 (c)	15.8 (c)	5.4 (b)	6.8 (e)	5.9 (b)

APPENDIX (Continued)

	United States	Germany	Japan	Netherlands	Canada	United Kingdom
Physician payment						
GPs	Fee-for-service; capitation; salary	Fee-for-service according to regional fee schedule	Fee-for-service according to point-fee schedule	Capitation for sickness-fund insured patients; fee-for-service for privately insured patients	Fee-for-service according to provincial fee schedule	Capitation, fees, and salary
Specialists	Fee-for-service; capitation; salary Medicare program uses the resource-based relative value scale to prospectively set reimbursement rates for outpatient physician services.[6]	Physicians in public hospitals are on salary; others paid fee-for-service according to regional fee schedule	Hospital-based physicians are on salary	Fee-for-service	Fee-for-service according to provincial fee schedule	Salary; fee-for-service
Hospitals						
Inpatient beds per 1,000 population						
1985	5.5	8.7	14.7	11.9	6.7	7.4
1996	4.0	9.6	16.2	11.2	5.1 (a)	4.5

Average length of stay (in days) for inpatient care						
1985	9.2	17.4	54.2	34.3	13.8	15.8
1996	7.8	14.3	43.7[7]	32.5	12.0	9.8
Hospital ownership	Nongovernmental nonprofit organizations: 59% state and local governments: 26% for-profit investor owned: 15%	Of total hospital beds: public hospitals: 51% nonprofit hospitals: 35% private hospitals: 14%	Slightly more than 80% of all hospitals and 70% of all hospitals beds are privately owned.	For-profit hospitals are prohibited; 85% of all hospitals are private not-for-profit institutions; 15% are public hospitals.	Nearly all hospitals are nonprofit entities run by community boards of trustees, voluntary organizations, or municipalities.	The NHS owns and operates more than 2,000 hospitals; there are also approximately 300 private hospitals, two-thirds of which are owned by for-profit organizations. Fewer than 10% of all acute care hospital beds are private.
Hospital payment	Fee-for-service; per diem; fee-per-case. The Medicare program uses the diagnosis-related group (DRG)-based Prospective Payment System that provides for fixed payment for specific medical cases.	Per diem rate hospital payment system to be replaced by mixed payment system with case fees, procedure fees and separate departmental per diem rates.	Hospitals paid a standard per diem rate	Fee-for-service	Fee-for-service	Fee-for-service; fee-per-case

189

	United States	Germany	Japan	Netherlands	Canada	United Kingdom
High-tech equipment						
MRIs per million population	16.0 (c)	5.7 (b)	18.8 (b)	3.9 (c)	1.7 (a)	3.4 (c)
Scanners per million population	26.9 (e)	16.4 (b)	69.7 (b)	9.0 (e)	8.1 (a)	6.3 (e)

Sources: OECD Health Data 98: A Comparative Analysis of 29 Countries. U.S. Health Care Financing Administration; Canadian Institute of Health Information; Ministry of Health and Welfare, Japan; World Bank.

Note: (a) 1997; (b) 1996; (c) 1995; (d) 1994; (e) 1993; (f) 1992; (g) 1991.

[1] Per capita expenditure is adjusted for purchasing power parities (PPPs). PPPs express the rate at which one currency should be converted to another to purchase the same set of goods and services in both countries.

[2] Infant deaths per 1,000 live births.

[3] This includes individuals who earn above the income limit for mandatory coverage under the sickness fund program (and who are therefore free to choose private insurance) but choose to be covered under the sickness fund insurance program.

[4] Medicare Part A pays for hospital care, limited nursing home care, home health care and hospice care. Part B covers physicians services and is financed by enrollee premiums and general tax revenues.

[5] Total expenditures on inpatient care; physicians' services; and pharmaceutical goods as a percentage of total health expenditures.

[6] Volume Performance Standards (VPS) set annual target growth rate of the volume of physician services under Medicare.

[7] This figure includes long-term care facilities as well. The ALOS for general hospitals in Japan is 33.7 days.

References and Bibliographic Entries

CHAPTER 1

Anderson, Odin. 1989. *The Health Services Continuum in Democratic States*. Ann Arbor, Mich.: Health Administration Press.

Chernichovsky, Dov. 1995. "Health System Reforms in Industrialized Democracies: An Emerging Paradigm." *The Milbank Quarterly* 73, no. 3.

Davis, Karen. 1990. Response to Bengt Jonsson's article in *Health Care Systems in Transition*. Paris: OECD.

Enthoven, Alain. 1990. "What Can Europeans Learn from Americans?" In *Health Care Systems in Transition*. Paris: OECD.

Evans, Robert G. 1986. "The Spurious Dilemma: Reconciling Medical Progress and Cost Control." *Health Matrix* 4, no. 1.

———. 1997. "Going for the Gold: The Redistributive Agenda behind Market-Based Health Care Reform." *Journal of Health Politics, Policy and Law* 22, no. 2.

Evans, Robert G., and Morris L. Barer. 1990. "The American Predicament." In *Health Care Systems in Transition*. Paris: OECD.

Henke, Klaus-Dirk. 1990. Response to Bengt Jonsson's article in *Health Care Systems in Transition*. Paris: OECD.

Hsiao, William. 1992. "Comparing Health Care Systems: What Nations Can Learn from One Another." *Journal of Health Politics, Policy and Law* 17, no. 4.

Iglehart, John. 1989. "American Business Looks Abroad." *Health Affairs* 8, no. 4.

Jonsson, Bengt. 1990. "What Can Americans Learn from Europeans?" In *Health Care Systems in Transition*. Paris: OECD.

Kirkman-Liff, Bradford. 1989. "Cost Containment and Physician Payment Methods in the Netherlands." *Inquiry* 26.

Klein, Rudolf. 1991. "Risks and Benefits of Comparative Studies: Notes from Another Shore." *The Milbank Quarterly* 69, no 2.

———. 1995. "Big Bang Health Care Reform—Does It Work?: The Case of Britain's 1991 National Health Service Reforms." *The Milbank Quarterly* 73, no. 3.

Light, Donald. 1997. "From Managed Competition to Managed Cooperation: Theory and Lessons from the British Experience." *The Milbank Quarterly* 75, no. 3.

Mechanic, David. 1995. "The Americanization of the British National Health Service." *Health Affairs* (Summer).

Morone, James. 1990. "American Political Culture and the Search for Lessons from Abroad." *Journal of Health Politics, Policy and Law* 15, no. 1.

Organization for Economic Cooperation and Development (OECD). 1987. *Financing and Delivering Health Care* (Social Policy Studies No. 4). Paris: Author.

———. 1994. *The Reform of Health Care Systems: A Review of Seventeen OECD Countries* (Health Policy Studies No. 5). Paris: Author.

———. 1996. *Health Care Reform: The Will to Change* (Health Policy Studies No. 8). Paris: Author.

Pfaff, Martin. 1990. "Differences in Health Care Spending across Countries: Statistical Evidence." *Journal of Health Politics, Policy and Law* 15, no. 1.

Reinhardt, Uwe. 1990. Response to Bengt Jonsson's article in *Health Care Systems in Transition*. Paris: OECD.

Saltman, Richard, and Josep Figueras (eds.). 1997. *European Health Care Reform*. Copenhagen: Regional Office for Europe, World Health Organization.

Scheil-Adlung, Xenia. 1998. "Steering the Health Care Ship: Effects of Market Incentives to Control Costs in Selected OECD Countries." *International Social Security Review* 51, no. 1.

CHAPTER 2

Aaron, Henry J. 1994. "Thinking Straight about Medical Costs." *Health Affairs* 13, no. 5.

———. 1996a. "End of an Era: The New Debate over Health Care Financing." *The Brookings Review* (Winter 1996).

———. 1996b. "Thinking about Health Care Finance: Some Propositions." In *Health Care Reform: The Will to Change* (OECD Health Policy Studies 8). Paris: OECD.

Aaron, Henry, and Robert D. Reischauer. 1998. " 'Rethinking Medicare Reform' Needs Rethinking." *Health Affairs* 17, no. 1.

Albert, Lynn. 1998a. "Market-Based Restructuring: Employers' Health Care Strategies." *Watson Wyatt Insider* 8, no. 7.

———. 1998b. "Unmanaged Competition: A Vehicle for Health-Care Market Reform?" *Watson Wyatt Insider* 8, no. 6.

American Association of Health Plans (AAHP). 1998. *Managed Care Facts*. Washington, D.C.: Author.

Anders, George. 1998. "Kaiser's Red Ink Signals Trouble for HMOs." *Wall Street Journal*, February 17.

Berenson, Robert. 1998. "Pay FFS to Primary Care MDs While Capitating Specialists." *Managed Care Facts, Trends, and Data: 1998–99*. Washington, D.C.: Atlantic Information Services.

Berwick, Donald. 1996. "Payment by Capitation and the Quality of Care." *New England Journal of Medicine* 335, no. 16.

Bindman, Andrew, Kevin Grumbach, Karen Vranizan, Deborah Jaffe, and Dennis Osmond. 1998. "Selection and Exclusion of Primary Care Physicians by Managed Care Organizations." *Journal of the American Medical Association* 279, no. 9.

Blendon, Robert J., Mollyann Brodie, and John Benson. 1995. "What Happened to Americans' Support for the Clinton Health Plan?" *Health Affairs* 14, no. 2.

Blendon, Robert J., Mollyann Brodie, John Benson, Drew Altman, Larry Levitt, Tina Huff, and Lary Hugick. 1998. "Understanding the Managed Care Backlash." *Health Affairs* 17, no. 4.

Blendon, Robert, Robert Leitman, Ian Morrison, and Karen Donelan. 1990. "Satisfaction with Health Systems in Ten Nations." *Health Affairs* 9, no. 2.

Bodenheimer, Thomas. 1996. "The HMO Backlash—Righteous or Reactionary?" *New England Journal of Medicine* 335, no. 21.

Bodenheimer, Thomas, and Kip Sullivan. 1998. "How Large Employers Are Shaping the Health Care Marketplace" (two-part series) *New England Journal of Medicine* 338, no. 14, and 338, no. 15.

Budetti, Peter. 1998. "Health Insurance for Children—A Model for Incremental Health Reform?" *New England Journal of Medicine* 338, no. 8.

Carnevale, Mary Lu. 1989. "Union Workers Begin Strike at Nynex, Bell Atlantic and Pacific Telesis Group." *Wall Street Journal,* August 7.

Carney, Eliza Newlin, and Marilyn Werber Serafini. 1998. "A Popular Legislative Prescription." *National Journal,* April 25.

Cooper, Philip F., and Barbara Steinberg Schone. 1997. "More Offers, Fewer Takers for Employment-Based Health Insurance: 1987 and 1996." *Health Affairs* 16, no. 6.

Crenshaw, Albert. 1989. "Health Care: The New Labor Battleground." *Washington Post,* August 8.

Davis, Karen. 1996. "Incremental Coverage of the Uninsured." *Journal of the American Medical Association* 276, no. 10.

The Economist. 1998a. "Health Care in America" (March 7).

———. 1998b. "Patients or Profits?" (March 7).

Ellwood, Paul M., and George D. Lundberg. 1996. "Managed Care: A Work in Progress." *Journal of the American Medical Association* 276, no. 13.

Employee Benefit Research Institute. 1995. Issue Brief No. 167 (November).

Enthoven, Alain C. 1993. "The History and Principles of Managed Competition." *Health Affairs* 12 (suppl.).

Enthoven, Alain C., and Richard Kronick. 1989. "A Consumer-Choice Health Plan for the 1990s." *New England Journal of Medicine* (two-part series) 320, nos. 2 and 15.

Enthoven, Alain C., and Sara J. Singer. 1994. "A Single-Payer System in Jackson Hole Clothing." *Health Affairs* 13, no. 1.

———. 1997. "Markets and Collective Action in Regulating Managed Care." *Health Affairs* 16, no. 6.

Fisher, Ian. 1998. "H.M.O. Premiums Rising Sharply, Stoking Debate on Managed Care." *New York Times,* January 11.

Freudenheim, Milt. 1989a. "A Health Care Taboo Is Broken." *New York Times,* May 8.

———. 1989b. "Calling for a Bigger U.S. Health Role." *New York Times,* May 30.

———. 1989c. "Debating Canadian Health `Model.' *New York Times,* June 29.

———. 1998a. "Companies Getting More Involved in Health Care." *New York Times,* April 9.

———. 1998b. "Exiting Medicare Is Not a Sure Solution for HMO Woes." *New York Times,* October 6.

————. 1998c. "(Loosely) Managed Care Is in Demand." *New York Times,* September 28.

————. 1998d. "Progress on Health Costs, But Nagging Woes Persist." *New York Times,* January 5.

Fronstin, Paul. 1998a. "Features of Employment-Based Health Plans." *EBRI Issue Brief* no. 201 (September).

————. 1998b. "Sources of Health Insurance and Characteristics of the Uninsured." *EBRI Issue Brief* no 204 (December).

Fronstin, Paul, and Craig Copeland. 1997. "Medicare on Life Support: Will It Survive?" *EBRI Issue Brief* no. 189 (September).

Fronstin, Paul, and Jennifer Hicks. 1998. "Confidence in Health Care at What Cost?" *EBRI Issue Brief* no. 199 (July).

Fubini, Sylvia, and Steve Bush. 1998. "The Provider as White Knight." *Healthcare Trends Report* 12, no. 9.

Fuchs, Victor. 1994. "The Clinton Plan: A Researcher Examines Reform." *Health Affairs* 13, no. 1.

————. 1997. "Managed Care and Merger Mania." *Journal of the American Medical Association* 277, no. 11.

Gawande, Atul, Robert Blendon, Mollyann Brodie, John Benson, Larry Levitt, and Larry Hugick. 1998. "Does Dissatisfaction with Health Plans Stem from Having No Choices?" *Health Affairs* 17, no. 5.

Ginsburg, Paul. 1998. "Health System Change in 1997." *Health Affairs* 17, no. 4.

Ginsberg, Paul, and Jon R. Gabel. 1998. "Tracking Health Care Costs: What's New in 1998?" *Health Affairs* 17, no. 5.

Ginsburg, Paul, and Jeremy Pickreign. 1996. "Tracking Health Care Costs." *Health Affairs* 15, no. 3.

Ginzberg, Eli. 1990. "Health Care Reform—Why So Slow?" *New England Journal of Medicine* 322, no. 20.

————. 1996. "The Health Care Market: Theory and Reality." *Journal of the American Medical Association* 276, no. 10.

————. 1997a. "Managed Care—A Look Back and a Look Ahead." *New England Journal of Medicine* 336, no. 4.

————. 1997b. "Managed Care and the Competitive Market in Health Care: What They Can and Cannot Do." *Journal of the American Medical Association* 277, no. 22.

————. 1998. "The Changing U.S. Health Care Agenda." *Journal of the American Medical Association* 279, no. 7.

Gold, Marcia, Robert Hurley, Timothy Lake, Todd Ensor, and Robert Berenson. 1995. "A National Survey of the Arrangements Managed-Care Plans Make with Physicians." *New England Journal of Medicine* 333, no. 25.

Goldstein, Amy, and Terry Neal. 1998. "Health Care Uproar Has Hill Scrambling." *Washington Post,* May 31.

Graig, Laurene A. 1993. *State Health Reform.* Washington, D.C.: Wyatt.

Hilzenrath, David. 1998a. "Disability Claims Rise for Doctors." *Washington Post,* February 16.

————. 1998b. "Large Firms Paying More for Health Care." *Washington Post,* January 7.

Iglehart, John K. 1992a. "Health Policy Report: The American Health Care System—Introduction." *New England Journal of Medicine* 326, no. 14.

———. 1992b. "Health Policy Report: Private Insurance." *New England Journal of
Medicine* 326, no. 25.

———. 1992c. "Health Policy Report: Managed Care." *New England Journal of
Medicine* 327, no. 10.

———. 1992d. "Health Policy Report: Medicare." *New England Journal of Medicine* 327, no. 20.

———. 1993a. "Health Policy Report: Medicaid." *New England Journal of Medicine*
328, no. 12.

———. 1993b. "Health Care Reform: The Labyrinth of Congress." *New England
Journal of Medicine* 329, no. 21.

———. 1994a. "Health Care Reform: The Role of Physicians." *New England Journal of Medicine* 330, no. 10.

———. 1994b. "Health Policy Report: The Struggle between Managed Care and
Fee-for-Service Practice." *New England Journal of Medicine* 331, no. 1.

———. 1994c. "Health Policy Report: Physicians and the Growth of Managed
Care." *New England Journal of Medicine* 331, no. 17.

———. 1995a. "Health Policy Report: Republicans and the New Politics of Health
Care." *New England Journal of Medicine* 332, no. 14.

———. 1995b. "Health Policy Report: Medicaid and Managed Care." *New England Journal of Medicine* 332, no. 25.

———. 1996. "Health Policy Report: The Struggle to Reform Medicare." *New
England Journal of Medicine* 334, no. 16.

———. 1997a. "Health Policy Report: Health Issues, The President, and the 105th
Congress." *New England Journal of Medicine* 336, no. 9.

———. 1997b. "Occasional Notes: Listening in on the Duke University Private
Sector Conference." *New England Journal of Medicine* 336, no. 25.

———. 1998. "Physicians as Agents of Social Control: The Thoughts of Victor
Fuchs." *Health Affairs* 17, no. 1.

———. 1999. "The American Health Care System—Expenditures." *New England
Journal of Medicine* 340, no. 1.

Ignagni, Karen. 1998. "Covering a Breaking Revolution: The Media and Managed
Care." *Health Affairs* 17, no. 1.

Jensen, Gail A., Michael A. Morrisey, Shannon Gaffney, and Derek K. Liston. 1997.
"The New Dominance of Managed Care: Insurance Trends in the 1990s." *Health
Affairs* 16, no. 1.

Henry J. Kaiser Family Foundation. 1998. *Trends and Indicators in the Changing
Health Care Marketplace.* Menlo Park, Calif.: Author.

Kassirer, Jerome. 1995. "Managed Care and the Morality of the Marketplace." *New
England Journal of Medicine* 333, no. 1.

———. 1997. "Is Managed Care Here to Stay?" *New England Journal of Medicine*
336, no. 1.

———. 1998. "Managing Care—Should We Adopt A New Ethic?" *New England
Journal of Medicine* 339, no. 6.

Klein, Rudolf. 1995. "Big Bang Health Care Reform—Does It Work?: The Case of Britain's 1991 National Health Service Reforms." *The Milbank Quarterly* 73, no. 3.

Kletke, P., D. Emmons, and K. Gillis. 1996. "Current Trends in Physicians' Practice Arrangements, from Owners to Employees." *Journal of the American Medical Association* 276.

Kuttner, Robert. 1998. "Must Good HMOs Go Bad?" *New England Journal of Medicine* (two-part series) 338, no. 21; and 338, no. 22.

Langreth, Robert. 1998. "After Seeing Profits from the Poor, Some HMOs Abandon Them." *Wall Street Journal,* April 7.

Levit, Katharine, and Cathy Cowan. 1991. "Business, Households, and Governments: Health Care Costs, 1990." *Health Care Financing Review* 13, no. 2.

Levit, Katharine, Cathy Cowan, Bradley Braden, Jean Stiller, Arthur Sensenig, and Helen Lazenby. 1998. "National Health Expenditures in 1997: More Slow Growth." *Health Affairs* 17, no. 6.

Light, Donald. 1998. "Is NHS Purchasing Serious? An American Perspective." *British Medical Journal* 316 (January 17).

Marmor, Ted. 1993. "The History of Health Care Reform." *Roll Call Health Care Policy Briefing* (July 19).

Mayer, Thomas R., and Gloria Gilbert Mayer. 1985. "HMOs: Origins and Development." *New England Journal of Medicine,* February 28.

McGinley, Laurie, and Jeanne Cummings. 1998. "Clinton Touts Plan to Make Health Care More Affordable for Elderly and Others." *Wall Street Journal,* March 18.

Mechanic, David. 1997. "Managed Care as a Target of Distrust." *Journal of the American Medical Association* 277, no. 22.

Neal, Terry. 1998. "Democrats Try to Take Health Care Reins on Managed Health Care Overhaul." *Washington Post,* April 9.

O'Keefe, Janet. 1992. "Health Care Financing: How Much Reform Is Needed?" *Issues in Science and Technology* VII, no. 3.

OECD. 1994. *The Reform of Health Care Systems: A Review of 17 OECD Countries* (OECD Health Policy Studies no. 5). Paris: Author.

———. 1996. *Health Care Reform: The Will to Change* (OECD Health Policy Studies no. 8). Paris: Author.

———. 1998. "Government Lags in Steps to Widen Health Coverage." *New York Times,* August 8.

Reinhardt, Uwe, E. 1994. "The Clinton Plan: A Salute to American Pluralism." *Health Affairs* (Spring, I).

———. 1995. *Managed Care, Capitation, and Managed Competition: A Brief Primer.* Princeton, NJ: Princeton University.

———. 1996a. "Economics." *Journal of the American Medical Association* 275, no. 23.

———. 1996b. "Health System Change: Skirmish or Revolution?" *Health Affairs* 15, no. 4.

———. 1997. "Wanted: A Clearly Articulated Social Ethic for American Health Care." *Journal of the American Medical Association* 278, no. 17.

Rodwin, Victor G. 1987. "American Exceptionalism in the Health Sector: The Advantages of Backwardness in Learning from Abroad." *Medical Care Review* 44, no. 1.

Samuelson Robert J. 1998. "HMO Backlash." *Washington Post,* March 4.

Serafini, Marilyn Werber. 1997a. "Oh, Yeah, the Uninsured." *The National Journal,* November 15.

———. 1997b. "Micromanaged Care." *The National Journal,* December 13.

———. 1998a. "The Deal Maker." *The National Journal,* February 14.

———. 1998b. "Insuring Early Retirees." *The National Journal,* March 14.

———. 1998c. "Medicare's Exodus." *The National Journal,* October 3.

———. 1998d. "A New Prescription." *The National Journal,* March 14.

Skocpol, Theda. 1995. "The Rise and Resounding Demise of the Clinton Plan." *Health Affairs* 14, no. 1.

Smith, Barbara Markham. 1997. "Trends in Health Care Coverage and Financing and Their Implications for Policy." *New England Journal of Medicine,* 337, no. 14.

Smith, Sheila, Mark Freeland, Stephen Heffler, David McKusick, and the Health Expenditures Project Team. 1998. "The Next Ten Years of Health Spending: What Does the Future Hold?" *Health Affairs* 17, no. 5.

Snyderman, Ralph. 1997. "The HMO Hazard: How the Quest for Short-Term Profits May Undermine Our Whole Health Care System." *Washington Post,* January 6.

Srinivasen, Srija, Larry Levitt, and June Lundy. 1998. "Wall Street's Love Affair with Health Care." *Health Affairs* 17, no. 4.

Starr, Paul. 1982. *The Social Transformation of American Medicine.* New York: Basic Books.

———. 1992. *The Logic of Health-Care Reform.* Grand Rounds Press.

Stevens, Rosemary. 1998. "Stickability and the Tax Exempt." *Hospitals and Health Networks* (July 5).

Stolberg, Sheryl Gay. 1998. "As Doctors Trade Shingle for Marque, Cries of Woe." *New York Times,* August 3.

Thorpe, Kenneth. 1997. "The Rising Number of Uninsured Workers: An Approaching Crisis in Health Care Financing" (Paper Prepared for the National Coalition on Health Care, October).

U.S. General Accounting Office (GAO). 1997a. *Employment-Based Health Insurance: Costs Increase and Family Coverage Decreases.* Washington, D.C.: U.S. Government Printing Office.

———. 1997b. *Private Health Insurance: Continued Erosion in Coverage Linked to Cost Pressures.* Washington, D.C.: U.S. Government Printing Office.

———. 1998a. Baby Boom Generation Presents Financing Challenges. Testimony before the Special Committee on Aging, U.S. Senate, March 9.

———. 1998b. *Health Insurance Standards: New Federal Law Creates Challenges for Consumers, Insurers, Legislators* (GAO/HEHS-98-67). Washington, D.C.: U.S. Government Printing Office.

———. 1998c. Retiree Health Insurance: Erosion in Retiree Health Benefits Offered by Large Employers. Testimony before the Subcommittee on Oversight, Committee on Ways and Means, U.S. House of Representatives, March 10.

Watson Wyatt Worldwide. 1997. *Survey Report on Employee Benefits 97/8.* Rochelle Park, NJ: Watson Wyatt Data Services.

Weiner, Jonathan, and Gregory de Lissovoy. 1993. "Razing a Tower of Babel: A Taxonomy for Managed Care and Health Insurance Plans." *Journal of Health Politics, Policy and Law* 18, no. 1.

————. 1995. *Competing Solutions: American Health Care Proposals and Interna-tional Experience*. Washington, D.C.: Brookings Institution.

Wyatt Company. 1990. *Management USA: Leading a Changing Work Force*. Wash-ington, D.C.: Author.

Yankelovich, Daniel. 1995. "The Debate that Wasn't: The Public and the Clinton Plan." *Health Affairs* 14, no. 1.

CHAPTER 3

Abel-Smith, Brian. 1984. *Cost Containment in Health Care: The Experience of Twelve European Countries (1977–1983)*. Luxembourg: Office of Official Publications of the European Communities.

————. 1985. "Who Is the Odd Man Out?: The Experience of Western Europe in Containing the Costs of Health Care." *Milbank Memorial Fund Quarterly/Health and Society* 63, no. 1.

————. 1988. "The Rise and Decline of the Early HMOs: Some International Ex-perience." *The Milbank Quarterly* 66, no. 4.

Abel-Smith, Brian, and Alan Maynard. 1979. *The Organization, Financing and Cost of Health Care in the European Community*. Luxembourg: Office of Official Pub-lications of the European Communities.

Altenstetter, Christa. 1985. "Hospital Policy and Resource Allocation in the Fed-eral Republic of Germany." In *Public Policy across Nations: Social Welfare in In-dustrial Settings*, ed. A. J. Groth and L. L. Wade. Greenwich, Conn.: JAI Press.

————. 1986. "German Social Security Programs: An Interpretation of Their De-velopment, 1883–1985." In *Nationalizing Social Security in Europe and America*, ed. D. E. Ashford and W. W. Kelley. Greenwich, Conn.: JAI Press.

————. 1987. "An End to the Consensus on Health Care in the Federal Republic of Germany?" *Journal of Health Politics, Policy and Law* 12, no. 3.

————. 1998. "From Solidarity to Market Competition? Values, Structure, Strat-egy in German Health Policy, 1883–1997." In *Health Care Systems in Transition: An International Perspective*, ed. Francis D. Powell and Albert F. Wessen. Thou-sand Oaks, Calif.: Sage Publications.

Anderson, Odin. 1989. *The Health Services Continuum in Democratic States*. Ann Arbor, Mich.: Health Administration Press.

Blanpain, Jan, L. Delesie, and H. Nys (eds.). 1978. *National Health Insurance and Health Resources: The European Experience*. Cambridge, Mass.: Harvard Univer-sity Press.

Blendon, Robert, Robert Leitman, Ian Morrison, and Karen Donelan. 1990. "Sat-isfaction with Health Systems in Ten Nations." *Health Affairs* 9, no. 2.

Brenner, Gerhard, and Dale A. Rublee. 1991. "The 1987 Revision of Physician Fees in Germany." *Health Affairs* 10, no. 3.

Covaleski, John. 1995. "U.S. Managed Care in Demand Overseas." *Best's Review Life/Health* (November).

Culyer, Anthony. 1990. "Cost Containment in Europe." In *Health Care Systems in Transition*. Paris: OECD.

Dahrendorf, Ralf. 1976. *Society and Democracy in Germany*. New York: W. W. Norton.

Donelan, Karen, Robert J. Blendon, Jon Benson, Robert Leitman, and Humphrey Taylor. 1996. "All Payer, Single Payer, Managed Care, No Payer: Patients' Perspectives in Three Nations." *Health Affairs* 15, no. 3.

The Economist. 1988. "Europeans Seek the Right Treatment" (July 16).

Edlin, Mari. 1997. "Pharmacy Benefits Go Global." *Managed Healthcare* (November).

Eichhorn, Siegfried. 1984. "Health Services in the Federal Republic of Germany." In *Comparative Health Systems: Descriptive Analyses of Fourteen National Health Systems,* ed. Marshall Raffel. University Park: Pennsylvania State University Press.

Engel, Styliani. 1996. "Managed Care European Style." *Managed Care Marketing* (January).

Evans, Robert G. 1990. "Tension, Compression, and Shear: Directions, Stresses and Outcomes of Health Care Cost Control." *Journal of Health Politics, Policy and Law* 15, no. 1.

Files, Ashley, and Margaret Murray. 1995. "German Risk Structure Compensation: Enhancing Equity and Effectiveness." *Inquiry* 32 (Fall).

Glaser, William. 1978. *Health Insurance Bargaining: Lessons for Americans.* New York: Gardner Press.

————. 1983. "Lessons from Germany: Some Reflections Occasioned by Schulenburg's Report." *Journal of Health Politics, Policy and Law* 8, no. 2.

————. 1984. "Hospital Rate Regulation: American and Foreign Comparisons." *Journal of Health Politics, Policy and Law* 8, no. 4.

Godt, Paul. 1987. "Confrontation, Consent and Corporatism: State Strategies and the Medical Profession in France, Great Britain and West Germany." *Journal of Health Politics, Policy and Law* 12, no. 3.

Goebel, Willi. 1989. "Reform of Health Services in the Federal Republic of Germany." *International Social Security Review* (April).

Goerke, Laszlo. 1996. "Introduction of Long-Term Care Insurance in Germany: An Economic Interpretation. *International Social Security Review* 47, no. 4.

Hamerow, Theodore (ed.). 1973. *The Age of Bismarck.* New York: Harper and Row.

Henke, Klaus-Dirk. 1986. "A 'Concerted' Approach to Health Care in Financing in the Federal Republic of Germany." *Health Policy* 6.

————. 1990a. Response to Bengt Jonsson's article in *Health Care Systems in Transition.* Paris: OECD.

————. 1990b. "The Federal Republic of Germany." In *Advances in Health Economics and Health Services Research* (Supplement #1: Comparative Health Care Systems). Greenwich, Conn.: JAI Press.

Henke, K., Margaret Murray, and Claudia Ade. 1994. "Global Budgeting in Germany: Lessons for the U.S." *Health Affairs* (Fall).

Hinrichs, Karl. 1995. "The Impact of German Health Insurance Reforms on Redistribution and the Culture of Solidarity." *Journal of Health Politics, Policy and Law* 20, no. 3.

Holborn, Hajo. 1969. *A History of Modern Germany 1840–1945.* Princeton: Princeton University Press.

Hurst, Jeremy W. 1991. "Reform of Health Care in Germany." *Health Care Financing Review* 12, no. 3.

Iglehart, John K. 1991a. "Germany's Health Care System" (pt. 1). *New England Journal of Medicine* 324, no. 7.

———. 1991b. "Germany's Health Care System" (pt. 2). *New England Journal of Medicine* 324, no. 24.

International Social Security Review. 1989. "Federal Republic of Germany: Major Reform of the Sickness Insurance Scheme" (February).

Jonsson, Bengt. 1990. "What Can Americans Learn from Europeans?" In *Health Care Systems in Transition.* Paris: OECD.

Kertesz, Louise. 1997. "The New World of Managed Care." *Modern Healthcare* (November 3).

Kirk, Don Lewis. 1996. "Germany Expands Long-Term Care Benefits." *Business Insurance* (May 20).

Kirkman-Liff, Bradford. 1990. "Physician Payment Reform and Cost-Containment Strategies in West Germany: Suggestions for Medicare Reform." *Journal of Health Politics, Policy and Law* 15, no. 1.

———. 1998. "Health Care Cost Containment in Germany." In *Health Care Systems in Transition: An International Perspective,* ed. Francis P. Powell and Albert F. Wessen. Thousand Oaks, Calif.: Sage Publications.

Klein, Rudolf. 1995. "Big Bang Health Care Reform: Does It Work? The Case of Britain's 1991 Reforms." *The Milbank Quarterly* 73, no. 3.

Knox, Richard. 1993. *Germany: One Nation with Health Care for All.* New York: Faukner and Gray.

Knox, Richard, and Christoph Straub. 1993. "Hospitals in Germany: A Case of 'More Is Less.'" In *Germany: One Nation with Health Care for All,* ed. Richard Knox. New York: Faukner and Gray.

———. 1998. "Germany Profits from Bill on Long-Term Care" (January).

Light, Donald W. 1985. "Values and Structure in the German Health Care Systems." *Milbank Memorial Fund Quarterly/Health and Society* 63, no. 4.

Lockhart, Charles. 1981. "Values and Policy Conceptions of Health Policy Elites in the United States, the United Kingdom and the Federal Republic of Germany." *Journal of Health Politics and Law* 6, no. 1.

Marketletter. 1997. "Disease Management and Health Insurance" (July 21).

Morone, James, and Janice Goggin. 1995. "Health Policies in Europe: Welfare States in a Market Era." *Journal of Health Politics, Policy and Law* 20, no. 3.

Mullan, Fitzhugh. 1998. "The 'Mona Lisa' of Health Policy: Primary Care at Home and Abroad." *Health Affairs* 17, no. 2.

Müller, Michael, and Klaus Uedelhofen. 1997. "New Directions for an Organized Health Care System in Germany." *European Management Journal* 15, no 6.

OECD. 1992. *The Reform of Health Care Systems: A Comparative Analysis of Seven OECD Countries.* Paris: Author.

———. 1997. *Economic Survey: Germany.* Paris: Author.

———. 1998. *OECD Health Data 98: A Comparative Analysis of 29 Countries.* Paris: Author.

Oloroso, Arsenio. 1995. "Caremark Heading Overseas with Managed Care Formula." *Crain's Chicago Business* (November 27).

Payer, Lynn. 1996. *Medicine & Culture.* New York: Henry Holt.

Penn, Merilyn. 1995. "Across the Ocean: Managed Care Reaches Europe." *Pharmaceutical Executive* (July).

Range, Peter Ross, and Robert Gerald Livingston. 1996. "The German Welfare Model That Still Is." *Washington Post,* August 11.

Reinhardt, Uwe. 1981a. "Health Insurance and Cost Containment Policies: The Experience Abroad." In *A New Approach to the Economics of Health Care,* ed. Mancur Olson. Washington, D.C.: American Enterprise Institute.

———. 1981b. "Health Insurance and Health Policy in the Federal Republic of Germany." *Health Care Financing* 3, no. 2.

———. 1990. "West Germany's Health Care and Health Insurance System: Combining Universal Access with Cost Control" (Report Prepared for the U.S. Bipartisan Commission on Comprehensive Health Care, Washington, D.C., June 25).

———. 1992. "Health Care uber Alles: How It Works in Germany." *Health Care Financial Management* 13, no. 4.

———. 1993. "Global Budgeting in German Health Care: Insights for Americans" (Paper presented to a conference on Managing Health Care Systems Under a Global Expenditure Limit, Washington, D.C., April).

———. 1994a. "Germany's Health Care System: It's Not the American Way." *Health Affairs* (Fall).

———. 1994a. "Medical Technology in Canada, Germany and the United States: An Update." *Health Affairs* (Fall).

———. 1998. "Uneasy Marks." *Hospitals & Health Networks* (May 5).

Saltman, Richard, and Josep Figueras. 1998. "Analyzing the Evidence on European Health Care Reform." *Health Affairs* 17, no. 2.

Scheil-Adlung, Xenia. 1998. "Steering the Healthcare Ship: Effects of Market Incentives to Control Costs in Selected OECD Countries." *International Social Security Review* 5, no. 1.

Schieber, George, Jean-Pierre Poullier, and Leslie M. Greenwald. 1991. "Health Care Systems in Twenty-Four Countries." *Health Affairs* 10, no. 3.

Scholte, Marianne, and Julia Doherty. 1998. "German Health System Slow to Change." *Managed Care Quarterly* 6, no. 2.

Schneider, Markus. 1991. "Health Care Cost Containment in the Federal Republic of Germany." *Health Care Financing Review* 12, no. 3.

Schwartz, Friedrich Wilhelm, and Reinhard Brusse. 1997. "Germany." In *Health Care Reform: Learning from International Experience,* ed. Chris Ham. Buckingham, England: Open University Press.

Spencer and Associates. 1989–1992. International Benefits Information Service. Chicaco.

Stevens, Carol. 1992. "Does Germany Hold the Key to U.S. Health Care Reform?" *Medical Economics* (January 6).

Starr, Paul. 1982. *The Social Transformation of American Medicine.* New York: Basic Books.

Stone, Deborah A. 1977. "Professionalism and Accountability: Controlling Health Services in the United States and West Germany." *Journal of Health Politics, Policy and Law* 2, no. 1.

———. 1979. "Health Care Cost Containment in West Germany." *Journal of Health Politics, Policy and Law* 4, no. 2.

———. 1980. *The Limits of Professional Power: National Health Care in the Federal Republic of Germany.* Chicago: University of Chicago.

————. 1991. "German Unification: East Meets West in the Doctor's Office." *Journal of Health Politics, Policy and Law* 16, no. 2.

————. 1995. "The Durability of Social Capital." *Journal of Health Politics, Policy and Law* 20, no. 3.

————. 1997. "The Doctor as Businessman: The Changing Politics of a Cultural Icon." *Journal of Health Politics Policy and Law* 22, no. 2.

Sullivan, Sean. 1993. "An America Perspective on the German Healthcare System." In *Health Care Policy and Politics: Lessons from Four Countries*, ed. Robert Helms. Washington, D.C.: AEI Press.

Suzman, Mark. 1996. "The Managed Care Remedy." *Financial Times*, September 9.

Swabey, John. 1990. "Social Security in the German Democratic Republic." *Benefits and Compensation International* (June).

U.S. General Accounting Office. 1991. *Health Care Spending Control: The Experience of France, Germany, and Japan* (GAO/HRD 92-9). Washington, D.C.: U.S. Government Printing Office.

————. 1993. *1993 German Health Reforms: New Cost-Control Initiatives* (GAO/HRD-93-103, July).

————. 1994a. *German Health Reforms: Changes Result in Lower Health Costs in 1993* (GAO/HEHS-95-27, December).

————. 1994b. *Prescription Drugs: Spending Control Initiatives from European Countries* (GAO/HEHS-94-30; GAO/HRD-93-103). Washington, D.C.: U.S. Government Printing Office.

————. 1994c. *Primary Care Physicians: Managing Supply in Canada, Germany, Sweden and the U.K.* (GAO/HEHS-94-111, May).

Van de Ven, Wynard. 1996. "Market-Oriented Health Care Reforms: Trends and Future Options." *Social Sciences and Medicine* 43, no. 5.

Watson Wyatt. 1998. *Benefits Report Europe*. Brussels: Author.

White, Joseph. 1995. *Competing Solutions: American Health Care Proposals and International Experience*. Washington, D.C.: Brookings Institution.

Wicks, Elliot. 1992. *German Health Care*. Washington, D.C.: Health Insurance Association of America.

Will, Wolfgang. 1989. "Health Reform in the Federal Republic of Germany." *Benefits and Compensation International* (August).

Wysong, Jere A., and Thomas Abel. 1990. "Universal Health Insurance and High-Risk Groups in West Germany: Implications for U.S. Health Policy." *The Milbank Quarterly* 68, no. 4.

Yakoboski, Paul, Jonathan Ratner, and David Gross. 1994. "The Effectiveness of Budget Targets and Caps in the German Ambulatory Care Sector." *Benefits Quarterly* (3d quarter).

Zollner, Detlev. 1982. "Germany." In *The Evolution of Social Insurance, 1881–1981*, ed. P. A. Kohler and H. F. Zacher. London: Frances Pinter.

CHAPTER 4

Abel-Smith, Brian. 1988. "The Rise and Decline of the Early HMOs: Some International Experiences." *The Milbank Quarterly* 66, no. 4.

————. 1992. "Cost Containment and New Priorities in the European Community." *The Milbank Quarterly* 70, no. 3.

Blanpain, Jan, Luc Delesie, and Herman Nys. 1978. *National Insurance and Health Resources: The European Experience.* Cambridge, Mass.: Harvard University Press.

Blendon, Robert J., Robert Leitman, Ian Morrison, and Karen Donelan. 1990. "Satisfaction with Health Systems in Ten Nations." *Health Affairs* 9, no. 2.

Cramb, Gordon. 1998. "Market Forces in Moderation." *Financial Times,* July 2.

de Roo, Aad. 1995. "Contracting and Solidarity: Market-Oriented Changes in Dutch Health Insurance Schemes." In *Implementing Planned Markets in Health Care,* ed. Richard B. Saltman and Casten von Otter. Buckingham: Open University Press.

Engel, Mari. 1997. "Pharmacy Benefits Go Global." *Managed Healthcare* (November).

Engel, Styliani. 1996. "Managed Care European Style: Part I." *Managed Care Marketing* (January).

Enthoven, Alain. 1990. "What Can Europeans Learn from Americans?" In *Health Care Systems in Transition.* Paris: OECD.

Frieden, Joyce. 1992. "Is Dutch Health Care a Model for the U.S. Health Care System?" *Business and Health* (May).

Graig, Laurene. 1994. "Dutch and British Systems Test Managed Competition." *Journal of International Compensation and Benefits* (July/August).

Greenberg, Warren. 1990. "Get Rid of Health Benefits on the Job." *Washington Post,* September 25.

————. 1993. "Lessons from the Netherlands." In *Health Care Policy & Politics,* ed. Robert B. Helms. Washington, D.C.: American Enterprise Institute.

Ham, Chris 1998. "Of Primary Concern." *Financial Times,* July 2.

Ham, Chris, and Mats Brommels. 1994. "Health Care Reform in the Netherlands, Sweden, and the United Kingdom." *Health Affairs* 13, no. 5.

Hamilton, Vivian. 1995. "Risk Selection: A Major Issue in Internal Markets." In *Health Care Reform through Internal Markets,* ed. Monique Jerome-Forget, Joseph White, and Joshua Wiener. Washington, D.C.: Brookings Institution.

IBIS Review. 1997. "Will Employers Become Involved with Health Care Costs?" (June).

Janssen, Richard, and Jan van der Made. 1990. "Privatization in Health Care: Concepts, Motives and Policies." *Health Policy* 14.

Jerome-Forget, Monique, Joseph White, and Joshua Wiener (eds.). 1995. *Health Care Reform through Internal Markets.* Washington, D.C.: Brookings Institution.

Jonsson, Bengt. 1990. "What Can Americans Learn from Europeans?" In *Health Care Systems in Transition.* Paris: OECD.

Kertesz, Louise. 1997. "The New World of Managed Care." *Modern Healthcare* (November).

Kirkman-Liff, Bradford. 1989. "Cost Containment and Physician Payment Methods in the Netherlands." *Inquiry* 26.

————. 1991. "Health Insurance Values and Implementation in the Netherlands and the Federal Republic of Germany: An Alternative Path to Universal Coverage." *Journal of the American Medical Association* 265, no. 10.

————. 1996. "Health Care Reform in the Netherlands, Israel, Germany, England and Sweden." *Generations* (June 22).

Klein, Rudolf. 1995a. "Big Bang Health Care Reform: Does It Work? The Case of Britain's 1991 Reforms." *The Milbank Quarterly* 73, no. 3.

————. 1995b. "Priorities and Rationing: Pragmatism or Principles?" *British Medical Journal* (September 23).

Lapre, Ruud. 1988. "A Change of Direction in the Dutch Health Care System?" *Health Policy* 10.

Life Insurance International. 1997. "Health Insurers Investigate Use of Smart Cards" (December).

Medical and Healthcare Marketplace Guide. 1997. "Managed Care and Pharmaceutical Benefit Management in Europe" (January).

Ministry of Health, Welfare and Sport. 1995. *Health Insurance in the Netherlands.* Rijswijk: Author.

Ministry of Welfare, Health and Cultural Affairs. 1988. *Changing Health Care in the Netherlands.* Rijswijk: Author.

————. 1989. *Health Insurance in the Netherlands.* Rijswijk: Author.

Mullan, Fitzhugh. 1998. "The 'Mona Lisa' of Health Policy: Primary Care at Home and Abroad." *Health Affairs* 17, no. 2.

Nicolai, J. P., and John Huff. 1994. "Health Care's Limits in Holland." *Wall Street Journal,* June 21.

OECD. 1992. *The Reform of Health Care Systems: A Comparative Analysis of Seven OECD Countries.* Paris: OECD.

Royal Embassy of the Netherlands. 1997. *Health Care in the Netherlands 1996.* Washington, D.C.: Author.

Saltman, Richard B., and Josep Figueras. 1998. "Analyzing the Evidence in European Health Care Reforms." *Health Affairs* (March/April).

Scheil-Adlung, Xenia. 1998. "Steering the Healthcare Ship: Effects of Market Incentives to Control Cost in Selected OECD Countries." *International Social Security Review* 51, no. 1.

Schut, Frederik. 1995. "Netherlands: Balancing Corporatism, Etatism, and Market Mechanisms." *Journal of Health Politics, Policy, and Law* 20, no. 3.

Spanjer, Marjanke. 1995. "Changes in Dutch Health Care." *The Lancet* (January 7).

Spencer and Associates. 1989–1998. International Benefits Information Service Briefing Service. Chicago.

van Barneveld, Erik Rene, C. J. A. van Vliet, and Waynand P. M. M. van de Ven. 1996. "Mandatory High-Risk Pooling: An Approach to Reducing Incentives for Cream Skimming." *Inquiry* 33 (Summer).

van de Ven, Wynand, and Frederik T. Schut. 1995. "The Dutch Experience with Internal Markets." In *Health Care Reform through Internal Markets,* ed. Monique Jerome-Forget, Joseph White, and Joshua Wiener. Washington, D.C.: Brookings Institution.

van de Ven, Wynand, Rene van Vliet, Erik Barneveld, and Leida Lamers. 1994. "Risk-Adjusted Capitation: Recent Experiences in the Netherlands." *Health Affairs* (Winter).

van Etten, G. M. 1990. "Recent Developments in Health Policy in the Netherlands" (Presentation given to World Health Organization seminar on Health Services in Europe in the 1990s, Prague, September 25–27).

CHAPTER 5

AARP. 1998. *Global Aging Report* 3, no. 3.

Abe, M. A. 1985. "Hospital Reimbursement Schemes: Japan's Point System and the United States' Diagnosis-Related Groups." *Medical Care* 23, no. 9.

Calhoun, Michael J. 1993. "The Japanese Health Care System in Perspective." In *Japan's Heath System: Efficiency and Effectiveness in Universal Care,* ed. Daniel Okimoto and Aki Yoshikawa. New York: Faulkner and Gray.

Campbell, John. 1996. "The Egalitarian Health Insurance System." In *Containing Health Care Costs in Japan,* ed. Naoki Ikegami and John C. Campbell. Ann Arbor: University of Michigan Press.

Campbell, Ruth. 1996. "The Three Minute Cure: Doctors and Elderly Patients in Japan." In *Containing Health Care Costs in Japan,* ed. Naoki Ikegami and John C. Campbell. Ann Arbor: University of Michigan Press.

Eisenstodt, Gale. 1992. "The Doctor's Margin." *Forbes* (November 23).

Employee Benefit Research Institute. 1989. "Japan Copes with Its 'Honorable Elders': Retirement and Health Benefit Systems in Japan." *EBRI Issue Brief* no. 92 (July).

Fujii, Mitsuru, and Michael Reich. 1988. "Rising Medical Costs and the Reform of Japan's Health Insurance System." *Health Policy* 9.

Government of Japan, Medical Care Insurance System Reform Council. 1997. *National Health Care for the 21st Century: Guidelines for Quality Medical Care and Ensuring an Insurance System for Everyone* (August 29).

Hashimoto, Masami. 1984. "Health Services in Japan." In *Comparative Health Systems,* ed. Marshall Raffel. University Park: Pennsylvania State University Press.

Horkitz, Karen. 1990. "International Benefits: Part One—Health Care." *EBRI Issue Brief* no. 106 (September).

Hsiao, William. 1996. "Afterword: Costs—the Macro Perspective." In *Containing Health Care Costs in Japan,* ed. Naoki Ikegami and John C. Campbell. Ann Arbor: University of Michigan Press.

Iglehart, John K. 1988a. "Japan's Medical Care System" (pt. I). *New England Journal of Medicine* 319, no. 12.

———. 1988b. "Japan's Medical Care System" (pt. II). *New England Journal of Medicine* 319, no. 17.

Ihara, Kazuhito. 1998. "Japan's Policies on Long-Term Care for the Elderly: The Gold Plan and the Long-Term Care Insurance." Unpublished paper.

Ikegami, Naoki. 1991. "Japanese Health Care: Low Cost through Regulated Fees." *Health Affairs* 10, no. 3.

———. 1996. "Overview: Health Care in Japan." In *Containing Health Care Costs in Japan,* ed. Naoki Ikegami and John C. Campbell. Ann Arbor: University of Michigan Press.

———. 1997. "Public Long-Term Care Insurance in Japan." *The Journal of the American Medical Association* 278, no. 16.

Ikegami, Naoki, and John C. Campbell. 1995. "Medical Care in Japan." *New England Journal of Medicine* 333, no. 19.

———. (eds.). 1996. *Containing Health Care Costs in Japan.* Ann Arbor: University of Michigan Press.

Jordan, Mary. 1997. "In Search of an Anesthetic Experience." *Washington Post,* November 24.

Katsumata, Yukiko. 1996. "Comparison of Health Expenditure Estimates between Japan and the United States." In *Containing Health Care Costs in Japan,* ed. Naoki Ikegami and John C. Campbell. Ann Arbor: University of Michigan Press.

Levin, Peter J., Jay Wolfson, and Hiroko Akiyama. 1987. "The Role of Management in Japanese Hospitals." *Hospital and Health Services Administration* (May).

Maher, Walter. 1990. "Back to Marketplace Basics." *Health Affairs* 9, no 1.

Marketletter. 1997a. "Health Care Reform Now Certain in Japan" (September 8).

———. 1997b. "Japan's Health Care Spending at Record" (November 24).

———. 1997c. "Japanese Health Insurance Move to Double Drug Cost" (May 19).

———. 1997d. "Japan Insurance Law Okd, with Revised Fees" (June 23).

Marmor, Theodore. 1992. "Japan: A Sobering Lesson." *Health Management Quarterly* (3d quarter).

Masuyama, Mikitaka, and John C. Campbell. 1996. "The Evolution of Fee-Schedule Politics in Japan." In *Containing Health Care Costs in Japan,* ed. Naoki Ikegami and John C. Campbell. Ann Arbor: University of Michigan Press.

Matsunaga, Yusuke. 1997. "Preparing for Old Age: The Challenge of Japan's Aging Society." *Nomura Research Institute Quarterly* (Spring).

Maurer, P. Reed. 1996. "Japanese Health Care Reform Is Coming." *Marketletter* (August 5).

Med Ad News. 1997. "Best Year Ever" (September).

Mitchell, Samuel. 1990. "Competitiveness and Excellence: Health Costs and U.S. Business." *Health Affairs* 9, no. 1.

Morishita, Kaoru. 1998. "Pension Reform Panel Skirts Key Funding Issues." *Nikkei Weekly,* October 19.

Murdo, Pat. 1989. "Challenges to Japan's Health Insurance System." *Japan Economic Institute Report,* no. 16A (April 21).

———. 1991. "Japanese Health-Care System No Panacea for Ailing U.S. Program." *Japan Economic Institute Report,* no. 25A (July 5).

Nikkei Weekly. 1997. "Health Care Changes Result in Fewer Outpatient Visits," November 3.

OECD. 1998. *OECD Health Data '98: A Comparative Analysis of 29 Countries.* Paris: Author.

Okimoto, Daniel, and Aki Yoshikawa. 1993. *Japan's Health System: Efficiency and Effectiveness in Universal Care.* New York: Faulkner and Gray.

Powell, Margaret, and Masahira Anesaki. 1990. *Health Care in Japan.* London: Routledge.

Reinhardt, Uwe. 1989. "Health Care Spending and Competitiveness." *Health Affairs* 8, no. 4.

———. 1990. "Health Care Woes of American Business: Reinhardt Responds." *Health Affairs* 9, no. 1.

Rodwin, Victor. 1994. *Japan's Universal Health Insurance System.* New York: Japan Society.

Sayle, Murray. 1998. "The Social Contradictions of Japanese Capitalism." *Atlantic Monthly* (June).

Schramm, Carl. 1990. "Living on the Short Side of the Long Run." *Health Affairs* 9, no. 1.

Social Insurance Agency. 1996. *Outline of Social Insurance in Japan.* Tokyo: Author.

Spencer and Associates. 1996–1998 passim. *International Benefits Information Service (IBIS).* Chicago.

Steslicke, William E. 1982. "Development of Health Insurance Policy in Japan." *Journal of Health Politics, Policy and Law* 7, no. 1.

———. 1989. "Health Care and the Japanese State." In *Success and Crisis in National Health Systems,* ed. Mark Field. New York: Routledge.

van Wolferen, Karel. 1989. *The Enigma of Japanese Power.* New York: Alfred Knopf.

Wall Street Journal. 1990. "Workplace: Working out Personnel Puzzles of the '90s," July 6.

White, Joseph. 1995. *Competing Solutions: American Health Care Proposals and International Experiences.* Washington, D.C.: Brookings Institution.

Wolfson, Jay, and Peter Levin. 1986. "Health Insurance, Japanese Style." *Business and Health* (May).

Yoshikawa, Aki. 1992. "Japan's Changing Health Care Environment" [Letter to Editor]. *Health Affairs* 11, no. 1.

———. 1993. "Doctors and Hospitals in Japan." In *Japan's Health System: Efficiency and Effectiveness in Universal Care,* ed. Daniel Okimoto and Aki Yoshikawa. New York: Faulkner and Gray.

Yoshikawa, Aki, and Osamu Utsunomiya. 1993. "Japan's Health Insurance System: From Cradle to Grave." In *Japan's Health System: Efficiency and Effectiveness in Universal Care,* ed. Daniel Okimoto and Aki Yoshikawa. New York: Faulkner and Gray.

Yoshikawa, Aki Jayanta Bhattacharya, and William B. Vogt. (eds.). 1996. *Health Economics of Japan.* Tokyo: University of Tokyo Press.

CHAPTER 6

Anderson, Odin W. 1989. *The Health Services Continuum in Democratic States: An Inquiry into Solvable Problems.* Ann Arbor, Mich.: Health Administration Press.

Andreopoulous, Spyros (ed.). 1975. *National Health Insurance: Can We Learn from Canada?* New York: John Wiley and Sons.

Barer, Morris. 1988. "Regulating Physician Supply: The Evolution of British Columbia's Bill 41." *Journal of Health Politics, Policy and Law* 13, no. 1.

Barer, Morris, and Robert G. Evans. 1986. "Riding North on a South-Bound Horse? Expenditures, Prices, Utilization and Incomes in the Canadian Health Care System." In *Medicare at Maturity,* ed. Robert G. Evans and Greg L. Stoddart. Calgary: University of Calgary Press.

Barer, Morris, Robert G. Evans, and Roberta J. Labelle. 1988. "Fee Controls As Cost Control: Tales from the Frozen North." *The Milbank Quarterly* 66, no. 1.

Barer, Morris, Jonathan Lomas, and Claudia Sanmartin. 1996. "Reminding our Ps and Qs: Medical Cost Controls in Canada." *Health Affairs* 15, no. 2.

Bell, Chaim, Matthew Crystal, Allan Detsky, Donald Redelmeier. 1998. "Shopping around for Hospital Services: A Comparison of the United States and Canada." *Journal of the American Medical Association* 279, no. 13.

Blomqvist, Ake. 1995. "Reforming Health Care: Canada and the Second Wave." In *Health Care Reform through Internal Markets: Experience and Proposals,* ed.

Monique Jerome-Forget, Joseph White, and Joshua Wiener. Washington, D.C.: Brookings Institution.

Brown, Barry. 1989. "How Canada's Health System Works." *Business and Health* (July).

Brown, Kenneth. 1989. "What We Can Learn from the Canadian Health Care System." In *Business, Work and Benefits: Adjusting to Change.* Washington, D.C.: Employee Benefits Research Institute.

Buske, Linda. 1998. "What's Covered? What's Not?" *Canadian Medical Association Journal* (July 14).

Canadian Institute for Health Information. 1998. "National Health Expenditure Trends, 1975–1998." www.ca.cihi.

Charles, Cathy, Jonathan Lomas, Nita Giacomini, Vandna Bhatia, and Victoria Vincent. 1997. "Medical Necessity in Canadian Health Policy: Four Meanings and a Funeral?" *The Milbank Quarterly* 75, no. 3.

Coutts, Jane. 1998a. "Ontario to Cap Use of New Drugs." *The Globe and Mail,* June 4.

DeCoster, Carolyn, and Marni Brownell. 1997. "Private Health Care in Canada: Savior or Siren?" *U.S. Department of Health and Human Services Public Health Reports* (July 17).

DeSantis, Solange. 1998. "Canadian Government's Health Care Cuts Create Private-Sector Opportunities." *Wall Street Journal,* March 25.

Dingwall, David. 1997. *Drug Costs in Canada.* Submitted to the House of Commons Standing Committee on Industry, March.

Evans, Robert G. 1975. "Beyond the Medical Marketplace: Expenditure, Utilization and Pricing of Insured Health in Canada." In *National Health Insurance,* ed. Spryos Andreopoulous. New York: Wiley.

———. 1984. *Strained Mercy: The Economics of Canadian Health Care.* Toronto: Butterworths.

———. 1986a. "Finding the Levers, Finding the Courage: Lessons on Cost Containment in North America." *Journal of Health Politics, Policy and Law* 11, no. 4.

———. 1986b. "The Spurious Dilemma: Reconciling Medical Progress and Cost Control." *Health Matrix* 4, no. 1.

———. 1987. "Hang Together or Hang Separately: The Viability of a Universal Health Care System in an Aging Society." *Canadian Public Policy* 12, no. 2.

———. 1988a. "Split Vision: Interpreting Cross-Border Differences in Health Spending." *Health Affairs* 7, no. 4.

———. 1988b. "We'll Take Care of It for You: Health Care in the Canadian Community." *Daedalus* (Fall).

———. 1990. "Tension, Compression, and Shear: Directions, Stresses and Outcomes of Health Care Cost Control." *Journal of Health Politics, Policy and Law* 15, no. 1.

———. 1995. "Managing Health Care Reform in Canada." In *Health Care Reform through Internal Markets: Experience and Proposals,* ed. Monique Jerome-Forget, Joseph White, and Joshua Wiener. Washington, D.C.: Brookings Institution.

———. 1998. "New Bottles, Same Old Wine: Right and Wrong on Physician Supply." *Canadian Medical Association Journal* (March 24).

Evans, Robert G., Jonathan Lomas, Morris Barer, Roberta Labelle, Catherine Fooks, Gregory Stoddart, Geoffrey Anderson, David Feeny, Amiran Gafni,

George Torrance, and William Tholl. 1989. "Controlling Health Expenditures—The Canadian Reality." *New England Journal of Medicine* 320, no. 9.

Evans, Robert G., and G. L. Stoddart (eds.). 1986. *Medicare at Maturity: Achievements, Lessons and Challenges.* Calgary: University of Calgary Press.

Government of Ontario. 1998. "Government and OMA Launch New Model for Delivering Patient Care." Press Release, May 26.

Gray, Charlotte. 1998. "The Private Sector Invades Medicare's Home Town." *Canadian Medical Association Journal* (July 28).

Greenberg, Larry M., Roger Ricklefs, and Mark Heinzl. 1997. "How Canada Endured Tough Choices to End a Damaging Recession." *Wall Street Journal,* December 26.

Ham, Faith. 1989. "Why Americans Like Canada's Health System." *Business and Health* (July).

Health Canada. 1998. *National Health Expenditures in Canada, 1975–1996.* www.hwc.ca.

Hurley, Jeremiah, Jonathan Lomas, and Laurie Goldsmith. 1997. "Physician Responses to Global Physician Expenditure Budgets in Canada: A Common Property Perspective." *The Milbank Quarterly* 75, no. 3.

Iglehart, John K. 1986a. "Canada's Health Care System." *New England Journal of Medicine* (3-pt. series) 315, no. 3.

———. 1986b. "Canada's Health Care System." *New England Journal of Medicine* 315, no. 12.

———. 1986c. "Canada's Health Care System." *New England Journal of Medicine* 315, no. 25.

———. 1989. "The United States Looks at Canadian Health Care." *New England Journal of Medicine* 321, no. 25.

———. 1990a. "Canada's Health Care System Faces Its Problems." *New England Journal of Medicine* 322, no. 8.

Jerome-Forget, Monique, Joseph White, and Joshua Wiener (eds.). 1995. *Health Care Reform through Internal Markets: Experience and Proposals.* Washington, D.C.: Brookings Institution.

Jerome-Forget, Monique, and Claude Forget. 1998. *Who Is the Master? A Blueprint for Canadian Health Care Reform.* Montreal: Institute for Public Policy.

Kane, Rosalie, and Robert Kane. 1985. "The Feasibility of Universal Long-Term Care Benefits: Ideas from Canada." *New England Journal of Medicine* 312, no. 21.

Katz, Stephen, Diana Verrilli, and Morris L. Barer. 1998. "Canadians Use of U.S. Medical Services." *Health Affairs* (January/February).

Kennedy, Mark. 1998. "Is It a Myth? Health Care Waiting Lists May Not Be Big Problem." *Windsor Star,* September 1.

Kirkey, Sharon. 1997. "Brokers Sell Swift U.S. Health Care." *Ottawa Citizen,* July 21.

Lindsay, Judy. 1998. "Big Spenders or Just Big Talkers?" *Vancouver Sun,* August 8.

Linton, Adam. 1990a. "The Canadian Health Care System: A Canadian Physician's Perspective." *New England Journal of Medicine* 322, no. 3.

———. 1990b. "Clinical Guidelines" (Presentation at the Ontario Medical Association Conference "How Green Is Your Grass?" Toronto, June 7–8).

Lomas, Jonathan. 1997. "Devolving Authority for Health Care in Canada's Provinces: Emerging Issues and Proposals." *Canadian Medical Association Journal* 156.

Lomas, Jonathan, Catherine Fooks, Thomas Rice, and Roberta Labelle. 1989. "Paying Physicians in Canada." *Health Affairs* 8, no. 1.

Lomas, Jonathan, John Woods, Gerry Veenstra. 1997. "Devolving Authority for Health Care in Canada's Provinces: An Introduction to the Issues." *Canadian Medical Association Journal* 156.

Marmor, Theodore, and Jerry Mashaw. 1990. "Canada's Health Insurance and Ours: The Real Lessons, The Big Choices." *American Prospect* (Fall).

Marshall, Robert. 1998. "The Health Report." *Macleans* (June 15).

Medical & Healthcare Marketplace Guide. 1997. "Pharmaceutical Retailing-Mail Service Pharmacy" (January).

Morone, James. 1990. "American Political Culture and the Search for Lessons from Abroad." *Journal of Health Politics, Policy and Law* 15, no. 1.

———. 1991. "A Different View of Queues in Ontario." *Health Affairs* 10, no. 3.

Morrison, Suzanne. 1998. "Primary Care Reform Not New." *Spectator,* May 27.

Mullan, Fitzhugh. 1998. "The 'Mona Lisa' of Health Policy: Primary Care at Home and Abroad." *Health Affairs* 17, no. 2.

National Forum on Health. 1997. "Canada Health Action: Building on the Legacy." Final Report of the National Forum on Health. Ottawa.

Neuschler, Edward. 1990. "Canadian Health Care: The Implications of Public Health Insurance." *HIAA Research Bulletin* (June).

Newhouse, Joseph P., Geoffrey Anderson, and Leslie L. Roos. 1988. "Hospital Spending in the United States and Canada: A Comparison." *Health Affairs* 7, no. 4.

Norton, James A. 1998. "Canadian Health Care at the Crossroads." *Managing Employee Health Benefits* 6, no. 3.

OECD. 1990. *Health Care Systems in Transition.* Paris: Author.

———. 1994. *The Reform of Health Care Systems.* Paris: Author.

———. 1995. *Internal Markets in the Making.* Paris: Author

Possehl, Suzanne. 1997. "Northern Plights." *Hospitals & Health Networks,* September 5.

Rachlis, Michael. 1995. "Defining Basic Services and Deinsuring the Rest: The Wrong Diagnosis and the Wrong Prescription." *Canadian Association Medical Journal* 152.

Rachlis, Michael, and Carol Kushner. 1989. *Second Opinion: What's Wrong with Canada's Health Care System and How to Fix It.* Toronto: Collins.

Ramsay, Cynthia, and Micheal Walker. 1998. *Critical Issues Bulletin: Waiting Your Turn: Hospital Waiting Lists in Canada.* 7th ed. Vancouver: Fraser Institute.

Regush, Nicholas. 1987. *Condition Critical: Canada's Health Care System.* Toronto: Macmillan of Canada.

Rice, Dorothy. 1998. "The Cost of Instant Access to Health Care." *Journal of the American Medical Association* 279, no. 13.

Schneider, Howard. 1998. "Budget Cuts Leave Canada's Prized Health Care System Ailing." *Washington Post,* July 2.

Sibbald, Barbara. 1998. "In Your Face: A New Wave of Militant Doctors Lashes Out." *Canadian Medical Association Journal* (June 2).

Spencer and Associates. 1998. International Benefits Information Service (May). Chicago.

Stevenson, H. Michael, A. Paul Williams, and Eugene Vayda. 1988. "Medical Politics and Canadian Medicare: Professional Response to the Canada Health Act." *The Milbank Quarterly* 66, no. 1.

Taylor, Malcolm. 1986. "The Canadian Health Care System 1974–1984." In *Medicare at Maturity*, ed. R. G. Evans and G. L. Stoddart. Calgary: University of Calgary Press.

Tuohy, C. J. 1986. "Conflict and Accommodation in the Canadian Health Care System." In *Medicare at Maturity*, ed. R. G. Evans and G. L. Stoddart. Calgary: University of Calgary Press.

Turner, Garth. 1996. "A Private Cure for Public Health Care." *Canadian Business* (January 1).

United States and Foreign Commercial Service. 1997. "Health Care Reform in Canada." *International Market Insight Reports*.

Vladek, Bruce. 1986. "American Perspective: If the War of 1812 Had Turned out Differently, Would There Now Be PPOs in Manitoba or Global Budgeting in Vermont?" In *Medicare at Maturity*, ed. R. G. Evans and G. L. Stoddart. Calgary: University of Calgary Press.

Warson, Albert. 1998. "Damage Control." *Modern Healthcare International* (May).

Watson Wyatt Worldwide. 1996. *Canadian Health/Dental Cost Management and Flexible Benefits Survey*. Toronto: Author.

Whitcomb, Michael E., and J. P. Desgroseilliers. 1992. "Primary Care Medicine in Canada." *New England Journal of Medicine* 326, no. 22.

White, Joseph. 1995. *Competing Solutions: American Health Care Reform Proposals and International Experience*. Washington, D.C.: Brookings Institution.

Wyatt Company. 1990. *Management USA—Leading a Changing Work Force*. Washington, D.C.: Author.

———. 1993. *1993 Survey of Group Benefit Plans Covering Salaried Employees of Canadian Employers*. Toronto: Author.

CHAPTER 7

Aaron, Henry, and William B. Schwartz. 1984. *The Painful Prescription*. Washington, D.C.: Brookings Institution.

———. 1990. "Rationing Health Care." In *Across the Board* (July/August).

Abel-Smith, Brian. 1985. "Who Is the Odd Man Out?: The Experience of Western Europe in Containing the Costs of Health Care." *Milbank Memorial Fund Quarterly/Health and Society* 63, no. 1.

———. 1992. "Cost Containment and New Priorities in the European Community," *The Milbank Quarterly* 70, no. 3.

Anderson, Odin W. 1989. *The Health Services Continuum in Democratic States: An Inquiry into Solvable Problems*. Ann Arbor, Mich.: Health Administration Press.

Blendon, Robert J., and Karen Donelan. 1989. "British Public Opinion on National Health Service Reform." *Health Affairs* 8, no. 4.

Charny, M., R. Klein, P. A. Lewis, and G. K. Tipping. 1990. "Britain's New Market Model of General Practice: Do Consumers Know Enough to Make It Work?" *Health Policy* 14.

Chernichovsky, Dov. 1995. "Health System Reforms in Industrialized Democracies: An Emerging Paradigm." *The Milbank Quarterly* 73.

Culyer, Anthony. 1989. Presentation at *Financial Post* Conference "Health Care in Canada," Toronto, June.

Curphy, Marianne. 1998. "Elderly Pay Price of Rising Medical Insurance Premiums." *Times of London,* June 13.

Day, Patricia, and Rudolf Klein. 1989. "The Politics of Modernization: Britain's National Health Service in the 1980s." *The Milbank Quarterly* 67, no. 1.

————. 1991. "Britain's Health Care Experiment." *Health Affairs,* 10, no. 3.

Dixon, Jennifer, and Nicholas Mays. 1997. "New Labour, New NHS?" *British Medical Journal* (December 20).

Eaglesham, Jean, and George Parker. 1997. "Medical Insurance: Over 60's Will Switch to NHS." *Financial Times* (July 3).

Earl-Slater, Alan. 1997. "Regulating the Price of U.K. Drugs: Second Thoughts after the Government's First Report. *British Medical Journal* (February 1).

The Economist. 1987. "Health: Thinking the Unthinkable." (August 22).

————. 1989a. "No Stopping Her." (February 4).

————. 1989b. "Short on Detail, Long on Questions." (February 25).

————. 1989c. "Still in Search of a Cure." (August 19).

————. 1989d. "A Tighter Prescription." (September 30).

————. 1990. "Treatment Suspended." (June 16).

————. 1991a. "Health Care Survey." (July 6).

————. 1991b. "Watered Down Medicine." (March 30).

————. 1992a. "Getting a Kick out of Reforms." (January 18).

————. 1992b. "Rolling Back the Private Sector." (June 6).

————. 1993. "Health Reforms: Seeing Double." (October 9).

————. 1995. "The Making of NHS Ltd." (January 21).

————. 1996a. "Safe in Whose Hands?" (October 26).

————. 1996b. "What's the Matter with the Health Reforms?" (May 25).

————. 1997a. "Coughing Up." (October 25).

————. 1997b. "Curing the NHS' Ills." (October 18).

————. 1997c. "How to Pay for the NHS." (March 15).

————. 1997d. "Prognosis: Poor." (May 3).

————. 1997e. "An Unhealthy Silence." (March 15)

————. 1998a. "Bevan's Baby Hits Middle Age." (July 4).

————. 1998b. "Waiting for Dobbo." (May 23).

Enthoven, Alain. 1990. "What Can Europeans Learn from Americans?" In *Health Care Systems in Transition.* Paris: OECD.

————. 1991. "Internal Market Reform of the British National Health Service." *Health Affairs* 10, no. 3.

Glennerster, Howard. 1995. "Internal Markets: Context and Structure." In *Health Care Reform through Internal Markets,* ed. Monique Jerome-Forget, Joseph White, and Joshua Wiener. Washington, D.C.: Brookings Institution.

————. 1996. "Population-Centered and Patient-Focussed Purchasing: The U.K. Experience." *The Milbank Quarterly* 74, no. 2.

————. 1998a. "The New NHS: Commentaries on the White Paper—From Command Economy to Demand Management." *British Medical Journal* (January 17).

————. 1998b. "The Next 10 Years: Analysis of the UK's National Health Service." *The Lancet* (July 4).

Hoare, Stephen. 1998. "Running Europe's Biggest Business." *Times of London*, June 23.

Jewell, Tony. 1997. "National Health Service under New Management." *The Lancet* (July 5).

Klein, Rudolf. 1991. "Risks and Benefits of Comparative Studies: Notes from Another Shore." *Milbank Quarterly* 69, no. 2.

————. 1995. "Big Bang Health Care Reform: Does It Work? The Case of Britain's 1991 NHS Reforms." *The Milbank Quarterly* 73, no. 3.

————. 1998. "Why Britain Is Reorganizing Its National Health Service—Yet Again." *Health Affairs* (July/August).

Lazarus, Ian. 1998. "In Search of Solutions: The United Kingdom Looks to U.S. Managed Care Tactics as It Enters an Era of Healthcare Reform." *Managed Healthcare* (May).

Light, Donald W. 1990a. "Bending the Rules." *Health Service Journal* 100, no. 5222.

————. 1990b. "Learning from Their Mistakes?" *Health Service Journal* 100, no. 5221.

————. 1991a. "Observations on the NHS Reforms: An American Perspective." *British Medical Journal* 303, no. 6802.

————. 1991b. "Perestroika for Britain's NHS." *The Lancet* 337, no. 874.

————. 1997. "From Managed Competition to Managed Cooperation: Theory and Lessons from the British Experience." *The Milbank Quarterly* 75, no. 3.

————. 1998. "Is NHS Purchasing Serious? An American Perspective." *British Medical Journal* (January 17).

Light, Donald, and Annabelle May. 1993. *Britain's Health System: From Welfare State to Managed Markets*. New York: Faulkner and Gray.

Lohr, Steve. 1988. "British Health Service Faces a Crisis in Funds and Delays." *New York Times*, August 7.

Lyall, Sarah. 1997a. "Blair Proposes to Overhaul National Health Service. *New York Times*, December 10.

————. 1997b. "For British Health System, Bleak Prognosis." *New York Times*, January 30.

Marmor, Theodore, and Rudolf Klein. 1986. "Cost vs. Care: America's Health Care Dilemma Wrongly Considered." *Health Matrix* 4, no. 1.

Maynard, Alan. 1990a. "The Case of Britain." *Health Policy* 15.

————. 1990b. "The United Kingdom." In *Advances in Health Economics and Health Services Research, Supplement 1: Comparative Health Systems*, ed. Jean-Jacques Rosa. Greenwich, Conn.: JAI Press.

————. 1993. "Competition in the U.K. National Health Service: Mission Impossible." *Health Policy*.

————. 1995. "Internal Markets and Health Care: A British Perspective." In *Health Care Reform through Internal Markets*, ed. Monique Jerome-Forget, Joseph White, and Joshua Wiener. Washington, D.C.: Brookings Institution.

Maynard, Alan, and Karen Bloor. 1996. "Introducing a Market to the United Kingdom's National Health Service." *New England Journal of Medicine* 334, no. 9.

Maxwell, Gary. 1995. "The Americanization of Britain's National Health Service." *Health Affairs* (Summer).

———. 1996. "Changes in Britain's Health Care." *Journal of the American Medical Association* 275, no 10.

Medical & Healthcare Marketplace Guide. 1997. "Private Healthcare in the United Kingdom."

Melcher, Richard, and Mark Maremont. 1989. "Thatcher's New Revolution." *Business Week* (May 1).

Murray, Ian. 1998a. "Half-Century Check-Up." *Times of London,* June 23.

———. 1998b. "Health Crusade Fails to Impress Professionals." *Times of London,* July 17.

OECD Health. 1995. *Internal Markets in the Making: Health Systems in Canada, Iceland, and the United Kingdom.* Paris: Author.

———. 1998. *OECD Health Data 98: A Comparative Analysis of 29 Countries.* Paris: Author.

Parston, Greg, and Laurie McMahon. 1998. "A Third Way? England Yes." *British Medical Journal* (January 17).

Pike, Alan. 1990a. "Health Managers Put Trust in Consultation." *Financial Times* (October 8).

———. 1990b. "Health Reforms under Attack." *Financial Times* (November 26).

———. 1990c. "Mood of Emergency on the Wards." *Financial Times* (March 10).

———. 1990d. "Perilous Path that Leads to NHS Reform." *Financial Times* (November 24).

———. 1990e. "State Hospitals Win Right to Control Their Finances." *Financial Times* (December 5).

———. 1990f. "U.K. Health Care." *Financial Times Survey* (January 29).

———. 1991a. "A Delicate Operation." *Financial Times* (March 28).

———. 1991b. "In Need of Care and Attention." *Financial Times* (July 30).

———. 1992. "Stitch-Up Treatment." *Financial Times* (September 13).

Potter, Christopher, and Janet Porter. 1989. "American Perceptions of the British National Health Service: Five Myths." *Journal of Health Politics, Policy and Law* 14, no. 2.

Prowse, Michael. 1989a. "Competitors in White Coats." *Financial Times* (August 22).

———. 1989b. "An Explosive Recipe." *Financial Times* (November 27).

———. 1990. "Buying on Behalf of Patients." *Financial Times* (February 28).

Robinson, Ray, and Julian LeGrand. 1995. "Contracting and the Purchaser-Provider Split." In *Implementing Planned Markets in Health Care,* ed. Micheal B. Saltman and Casten von Otter. Buckingham: Open University Press.

Rogaly, Joe. 1989. "The Doctors Carve up the Tories." *Financial Times* (October 20).

Rule, Sheila. 1990. "Quite Enough of Thatcher." *New York Times,* April 8.

Saltman, Richard, and Josep Figueras. 1998. "Analyzing the Evidence on European Health Care Reforms." *Health Affairs* (March/April).

Saltman, Richard, and Casten von Otter. 1995. *Implementing Planned Markets in Health Care.* Buckingham: Open University Press.

Scheil-Adlung, Xenia. 1998. "Steering the Healthcare Ship: Effects of Market Incentives to Control Costs in Selected OECD Countries." *International Social Security Review* 51, no. 1.

Smee, Clive. 1995. "Self-Governing Trusts and GP Fundholders: The British Experience." In *Implementing Planned Markets in Health Care,* ed. Richard Saltman and Casten von Otter. Buckingham: Open University Press.

Smith, David. 1998. "Charging Is the Only Cure for a Sickly NHS." *Times of London,* June 28.

Smith, Richard. 1998. "New Government, Same Narrow Vision." *British Medical Journal* (February 28).

Spencer and Associates. 1998. *International Benefits Information Service.* "Mini-Profile: UK" (April). Chicago.

———. 1997–1998. International Benefits Information Service. Chicago.

Terry, Derek, and R. Starbridge. 1997. "Industry Sector Analysis: U.K. Healthcare Service." American Embassy in London.

Timmons, Nicholas. 1998. "The NHS Today," and "New Pill to Treat a Recurring Headache." *Financial Times* (July 2).

———. 1999. "U.K. Learns from Others on Reform of Care for the Elderly." *Financial Times* (March 4).

U.K. Department of Health. 1989. *Working for Patients.* London: Her Majesty's Stationary Office.

U.K. Office of Fair Trading. 1998. *Health Insurance* (May).

Weiner, Jonathan P., and David M. Ferriss. 1990. "GP Budget Holding in the United Kingdom: Learning from American HMOs." *Health Policy* 16.

White, Joseph. 1995. *Competing Solutions: American Health Care Proposals and International Experience.* Washington, D.C.: Brookings Institution.

Willets, David. 1989. "The British Public and the Debate over the National Health Service." *Health Affairs* 8, no. 4.

Willman, John. 1992. "New Structure Expected to Manage NHS." *Financial Times* (August 21).

CHAPTER 8

Abel-Smith, Brian. 1988. "The Rise and Decline of the Early HMOs: Some International Experiences." *The Milbank Quarterly* 66, no. 4.

———. 1992. "Cost Containment and New Priorities in the European Community." *The Milbank Quarterly* 70, no. 3.

Bosworth, Barry, and Gary Burtless. 1997. "Budget Crunch: Population Aging in Rich Countries." *The Brookings Review* (Summer).

Buchanan, Allen. 1998. "Managed Care: Rationing without Justice, But Not Unjustly." *Journal of Health Politics, Policy and Law* 23, no. 4.

Fuchs, Victor R. 1991. "National Health Insurance Revisited." *Health Affairs* 10, no. 4.

Ginzberg, Eli. 1998. "U.S. Health System Reform in the Early 21st Century." *Journal of the American Medical Association* 280, no. 17.

Ikegami, Naoki. 1991. "Japanese Health Care: Low Cost through Regulated Fees." *Health Affairs* 10, no 3.

Klein, Rudolf. 1991. "Risks and Benefits of Comparative Studies: Notes from Another Shore." *The Milbank Quarterly* 69, no. 2.

Luesby, Jenny. 1998. "Healthcare Reforms Hit Japan's Prescription Drugs Market." *Financial Times* (September 24).

Morone, James A., and Janice M. Goggin. 1995. "Health Policies in Europe: Welfare States in a Market Era." *Journal of Health Politics, Policy and Law* 20, no. 3.

Reinhardt, Uwe. 1994. "Germany's Health Care System: It's Not the American Way." *Health Affairs* 13, no. 4.

———. 1997. "Wanted: A Clearly Articulated Social Ethic for American Health Care." *Journal of the American Medical Association* 278, no. 17.

Saltman, Richard B., and Josep Figueras. 1998. "Analyzing the Evidence on European Health Care Reforms." *Health Affairs* (March/April).

Scheil-Adlung, Xenia. 1998. "Steering the Healthcare Ship: Effects of Market Incentives to Control Costs in Selected OECD Countries." *International Social Security Review* 51, no. 1.

Starr, Paul. 1992. "The Ideological War over Health Care." *New York Times*, February 4.

White, Joseph. 1995. *Competing Solutions: American Health Care Proposals and International Experience.* Washington, D.C.: Brookings Institution.

Wilsford, David. 1995. "States Facing Interests: Struggles over Health Care Policy in Advanced, Industrial Democracies." *Journal of Health Politics, Policy and Law* 20, no. 3.

Index